QIGONG
—— FOR ——
MULTIPLE
SCLEROSIS

of related interest

Managing Depression with Qigong
Frances Gaik
ISBN 978 1 84819 018 4

Chinese Medical Qigong
Editor in Chief: Tianjun Liu
Associate Editor in Chief: Kevin W Chen
ISBN 978 1 84819 023 8

Traditional Chinese Medicine Approaches to Cancer
Harmony in the Face of the Tiger
Henry McGrath
ISBN 978 1 84819 013 9

QIGONG

—— FOR ——

MULTIPLE
SCLEROSIS

Finding your feet again

Nigel Mills

SINGING DRAGON
London and Philadelphia

First published in 2010
by Singing Dragon
an imprint of Jessica Kingsley Publishers
116 Pentonville Road
London N1 9JB, UK
and
400 Market Street, Suite 400
Philadelphia, PA 19106, USA

www.singing-dragon.com

Copyright © Nigel Mills 2010
Photography by Paulyne Skipsey

Library of Congress Cataloging in Publication Data
A CIP catalog record for this book is available from the Library of Congress

British Library Cataloguing in Publication Data
A CIP catalogue record for this book is available from the British Library

ISBN 978 1 84819 019 1

Printed and bound in Great Britain

CONTENTS

ACKNOWLEDGEMENTS

The development of the approach outlined in this book would not have been possible without three sets of people: first, the people I have worked with, who were experiencing the condition of multiple sclerosis (MS). I am continually amazed at the resilience and inner strength of people who face MS. I was particularly impressed by the commitment and perseverance of the people who participated in the programme and I was pleased to share in their progress.

Second, the development of this programme would not have been possible without my own experience of some excellent teachers of qigong. I would like to acknowledge particularly my first teacher Simon Carey-Morgan, who helped to design the initial programme and who undertook some of the initial individual training sessions. I have also benefited from some inspirational training in qigong from a range of other teachers including Brian Cooper; Bruce Frantzis; Daverick Leggett; Dek Leverton and, in more recent years, Zhixing Wang. I cannot claim to be an authorized teacher of any one qigong school or style. The final programme described in this book, reflects a personal selection of some qigong strategies, drawn from a broad range of sources, that I have found are usable by, and useful for, people with MS.

Third, I would like to thank those people who supported the research programme and scientific evaluation of the initial programme. The research study would not have been possible without the support and funding of the MS Research Trust and the statistical expertize of Janet Allan who carried out the analysis of the data.

Disclaimer

The techniques and practices described in this book are not intended to be used as a substitute for professional medical treatment and care. The book is intended to supplement any medical treatment being received. The book is also intended to supplement training from a recognized qigong instructor and is intended as a reference guide to complement 'live' instruction. If the reader undertakes any of the exercises, responsibility must lie solely with the reader.

Chapter 1

WHAT IS QIGONG AND WHY SHOULD IT BE USEFUL FOR MS?

What is qigong?

Qigong is a way of being.

Being soft, yet strong.

Qigong is a way of breathing.

Breathing deeply, yet calmly.

Qigong is a way of standing.

Alert, yet relaxed.

Qigong is...

A way of moving

A way of opening

A way of closing

A way of grounding

A way of giving

A way of receiving

A way of awakening

A way of healing.

How is it achieved?

By standing, in a certain way.

By breathing, in a certain way.

By stretching, in a certain way.

By bringing your awareness into your body, in a certain way.

By extending your awareness below your feet.

By learning how to move, in a certain way.

By letting go.

Through cultivating compassion for your body.

Through allowing yourself to be nourished by qi.

What is qi?

Qi is beyond words. The words are, however, attempted throughout the course of this book.

Where does qigong come from?

Qigong was developed as a means of achieving health and longevity in ancient China. Jahnke (2002) describes how qigong is first referred to in an ancient text called 'The Yellow Emperor's Classic Book of Medicine' (Ni 1995). This text was originally published around 300 BCE and contains some practical advice on to how to achieve health and live a long life. The material in this ancient text is presented as a form of dialogue between an apprentice 'Huang Ti' and his master 'Qibo'. Qibo instructs his apprentice as to how people in 'ancient' times lived well into their hundreds, without showing the usual signs of ageing. Qibo says that this is because:

> They formulated and utilized practices such as Dao Yin (the ancient word for qigong), including gentle body movements, self-applied massage, breath practice to promote qi flow, and meditation to harmonize themselves with nature and the universe. They lived a natural life of balanced diet, sufficient rest, avoidance of the effects of stress on body and mind and careful refraining from over-indulgence. They purposely maintained well-being in harmony with the body, mind, and spirit – it is no surprise that they lived in health over one hundred years. (Jahnke 2002)

The fact that in 300 BCE, the writer was referring to practices that were then considered from 'ancient times', indicates that the practice of qigong has been in existence for some considerable time! We can see from this ancient text then that the use of gentle body movements, self-applied massage, breath practice and meditation were, even then, the essential components of qigong. Each of these components will be introduced to some extent in this book.

How is qigong related to tai chi?

Tai chi is a relatively new development of qigong. Tai chi embodies the basic principles of alignment, posture and breathing that have been developed through qigong. However, tai chi takes these basic principles and uses them in the context of more complex patterns of almost dance-like movement. The patterns or 'forms' are said to have often been inspired by the study of nature, in particular the movements of animals.

Some of the forms were designed to develop abilities of self-defence, as used in the martial arts. Other forms were used to facilitate spiritual development:

> To lead the player from body to mind to spirit, and eventually back to the great void to merge with the cosmos.
> (Clark 2000)

However, the complex pattern of movements, called a 'form', that one is expected to learn in tai chi is quite taxing for the most able-bodied of people. It would be unrealistic to expect the average person who suffers from multiple sclerosis (MS) to develop the co-ordination, concentration and spatial awareness to initially learn a complex 'form' of tai chi.

Therefore in this book we will be focusing on the fundamental principles that underlie tai chi, referred to as 'qigong'. These principles include the cultivation of relaxed breathing, correct alignment of posture, slow and graceful movement, and meditation.

If, after following some of the exercises in this book, you are inspired to go and learn the 'forms' of tai chi, then you will usually find a tai chi class in a town nearby.

Many people find that the exercises of qigong open up such a world of inner movement and energy awareness, that they feel content to stay with the exercises of qigong and not embark on the more complex movements of a tai chi form. There are therefore an increasing number of classes just for 'qigong'.

My personal experience is that the more years I practise (currently 18 years) the more I come to realize that 'less is definitely more'. One of the fascinating aspects of qigong is that you can practise the same basic movement for many years and continue to develop a different awareness of your health and your energy through that same movement.

There is, to my mind, a danger of learning too many different movements and different patterns. There is a danger that you will acquire them like badges, moving from one to the next, without fully experiencing the development of health and energy that can be brought about from a focused practice of just one or two techniques.

This book, therefore, will not bombard you with a multitude of different 'things to do', but will instead attempt to transmit some basic, but powerful, principles as to how to help your body's own natural healing forces come to the fore.

Cultivation of qigong 'attitude'

If I am on a less than good day, I can draw energy and strength from sitting quietly and evaluating what I require. (Comment from participant in the research study)

The attitude with which you embark on qigong can be vitally important. One of the fundamental principles underlying qigong is that you need to trust that your body knows how to heal itself. In our Western culture we are particularly prone to try and 'sort things out'. Our minds are very good at creating lists of things to do and making arrangements, not to mention inventing motor cars and spaceships and tumble dryers. However, in the practice of qigong the mind has to take on a different skill, that is the skill of standing aside and allowing healing to occur.

Why should qigong be good for MS?

Qigong presents itself as a potentially very useful self-help approach for MS for the following reasons:

- People with MS often feel that their body is 'out of control' and 'alien'. Qigong cultivates a feeling of compassionate ownership of the body.

- People with MS often lose confidence in their ability to walk or carry out certain movements. Qigong slows down the process of walking and the process of movement so that the mind has sufficient time to enter the body and carry out desired movements in a more unified way.

- People with MS sometimes fear falling over, due to difficulties with balance. Qigong improves balance and reduces the likelihood of falling.

- People with MS often feel stressed and agitated. Qigong teaches a way of reducing nervous excitation and cultivating calm.

- People with MS often feel helpless and feel that there is nothing they can do to help their condition. Qigong encourages a sense of empowerment.

- Qigong helps you to 'find your feet again'.

Most of the practical aspects of the programme are taught in Chapters 5 and 6. Before launching into the practical aspects of the programme, however, I would like to provide some detail about how this self-help programme came to be independently validated at a UK-based National Health Service facility.

Chapter 2

THE RESEARCH STUDY

Qigong has given me an awareness of my body movements which had been unco-ordinated, even clumsy, and are now smoother and more relaxed. (Comment from participant in the research study)

The inspiration for this book came from a research study that was initially carried out in 1998 and 1999 and the material subsequently developed over the following years.

At that time I was employed as a clinical psychologist in the UK National Health Service, working in what is known as 'health psychology'. Health psychology involves trying to help people with a physical condition cope better, and improve their quality of life by using psychological strategies.

Listening to the stories of many of my clients with multiple sclerosis (MS) I noticed an enormous variation in the amount of physical exercise that people took and their attitude as to whether exercise was beneficial or detrimental. Some people with MS told me they had been advised not to engage in any exercise as it might make the condition worse. Other clients told me they had been advised to increase the amount of exercise they did. I turned to the research literature to see if there were any clear guidelines being recommended at that time. I found what I was looking for in an article by Petajan and White (1999), a neurologist and a sports scientist, who had that very year carried out a review of the scientific evidence concerning the role of physical exercise for people with MS. The authors also described how people with MS had traditionally been advised to avoid exercise, for fear that it could exhaust the patient and exacerbate the disease. Some people with MS also noticed that their symptoms are worse when they become hot, a condition known as thermo-sensitivity. The body's core temperature increases during exercise and can lead to a temporary worsening of symptoms.

However, if no exercise at all is undertaken then the muscles become weak and all the other problems of an excessively sedentary lifestyle develop. These may include obesity, cardiovascular problems, increased risk of depression and further fatigue due to lack of fitness. Petajan and White concluded that certain forms of exercise were, in fact, beneficial to people with MS as long as the exercise was designed to: 'Activate working muscles, but avoid overload that resulted in conduction block.'

Their review of the literature concluded that future research should explore the possible benefit of gentle mind–body exercise systems, which are not likely to overload the muscles and not likely to result in thermo-sensitivity. This recommendation stood out for me in bright lights. In my own personal life, one of the main things that kept me sane was my own practice of the mind–body exercise systems of qigong.

I began to think through the options. Should I be recommending to my clients that they learn qigong? I knew from my own experience that qigong classes were few and far between and often involved considerable travel. Tai chi classes were more readily available. However, having attended many different tai chi classes myself, when I envisaged some of my clients trying to keep up with the pace of such classes, I realized such an expectation was unrealistic. I recognized that the complex 'forms' attempted in a typical tai chi class would not be manageable by a large number of people with MS.

I then began to contemplate whether it would be possible for me to incorporate some of the principles of balance, movement breathing and mediation of qigong into my own sessions with clients. However, when I began to envisage this more clearly I could see that some clients may think it highly inappropriate; they had been referred to a psychologist to help with stress levels and were being asked to do weird movements in a small room. I quickly began to contemplate lots of professional problems arising and the possible disciplinary procedures that may be lurking on the horizon.

I contemplated how difficult it is for something outside the remit of normal professional practice services to become introduced into a traditional clinical setting. Here was an intervention that was being specifically recommended by medical scientists as worthy of exploration, yet how on earth would such an intervention come to be evaluated? I talked the issue through with my manager at that time, who encouraged me to submit an application to the Hospital Research and Ethics Committee for a research proposal. I therefore drew up a research plan entitled: 'An evaluation of qigong to help symptom management for people with multiple sclerosis.'

Many months later I was called to a room, which had a very long table and approximately 15 people sitting around it. This was the Hospital Research and Ethics Committee. The proposal was gone through with a fine tooth comb, looking at all the possible risks that may happen to a patient engaged in a qigong exercise programme. The panel were finally convinced that the level of risk was minimal and we were allowed to proceed to apply for research funding.

The Hospital Research and Ethics Committee were also impressed that, unlike many other 'alternative' therapies, that some of the principles of qigong and tai chi had already been substantially researched and the results published in reputable medical journals. Two studies were particularly relevant, one by

Jacobson *et al.* (1997) and one by Wolf *et al.* (1997). Both of these studies had shown that frail elderly people significantly improved their balance, and reduced their number of accidental falls, after putting into practice some of the principles of balance and movement taught in qigong and tai chi.

The improvement of balance for people with MS is very important. People with MS are very prone to falling over and incurring serious injury from the fall. This has been documented in a recent study by Peterson, Cho and van Kock (2008) who found that 50 per cent of a large sample of people with MS reported injurious falls.

I approached an organization called the MS Research Trust for funding to help us evaluate the study. The MS Research Trust were very interested in the idea and very helpful in their comments. After completing another detailed form on the aim and format of our proposed research, we were finally successful in being given a small grant. This meant that we could employ a researcher to evaluate independently the progress of people completing the programme. We recruited a doctoral level researcher from the University of Sussex called Janet Allen. Janet had already worked for some major drug companies and was very experienced in the design of research in the health field.

We were also able to fund some expert consultation to the study and some practical sessions from my own qigong teacher at that time, Simon Carey-Morgan. In addition to being a qigong instructor, Simon was also an acupuncturist and lecturer at the International College of Oriental Medicine in East Grinstead. He was, therefore, able to provide further insights from his knowledge of Chinese medicine.

Simon advised that the most essential aspects of qigong that were likely to help people with MS would be some of the basic principles underlying posture and movement. We agreed that it would be unrealistic to expect people with MS to master complex sequences of movement.

We wanted the programme to be realistic in terms of its likelihood of being able to be completed by people with MS. We also wanted it to target some of the particular problems faced by people with MS, in particular, problems with balance, problems with walking, muscle spasms, stiffness in joints, and numbness in fingers and feet. We also wanted the programme to be easily accessible and reproducible by other researchers and other teachers of qigong. We therefore decided to create a programme based on a range of basic qigong exercises that are broadly known and commonly used in qigong classes.

We carried out some pilot work, before commencing the main study, to ascertain what sort of exercises would be manageable by people with MS. This pilot work was very useful, as it showed us how we were initially too ambitious in the range and complexity of exercises that we used. Readers who are familiar with the names of some qigong exercises may be interested to know, for example, that the exercise 'cloud hands' (see Frantzis 2007 for a typical version) was much too difficult for most of the people with MS whom we worked with.

Furthermore the tendency to develop 'tai chi knee' (discomfort in the knee after practising particular tai chi and qigong exercises that involve twisting the body above the knee whilst keeping the feet still) was much more of a risk in people with MS.

Another factor which became clear was that many people with MS cannot stand for very long, if at all. The exercise programme therefore needed to contain some exercises that could be carried out whilst sitting.

Finally, many people with MS approached the exercises with some considerable anxiety as to whether they would be able to carry them out. This anxiety impeded their performance. We found that their performance improved if we first of all found a way of helping the person to feel safe and relaxed.

In summary, we realized that in designing the programme we needed to take the following issues into account:

- People with MS often have cognitive difficulties, which manifest as difficulties in concentration, co-ordination, and difficulties in memory. The exercise programme therefore needed to focus on a few simple but effective exercises, which would be fairly easy to remember and not too complex.

- People with MS often experience fatigue. The exercise programme could not be too tiring or too long.

- The exercise programme should avoid those exercises that involve lateral twisting above the knee whilst keeping the feet still.

- The exercise programme needed to include some exercises that could be carried out whilst sitting, but still have the aim of improving balance and walking ability.

- The exercise programme needed to include a way of helping the participant to feel safe and calm.

We searched for pre-existing publications on tai chi and qigong that described an approach that met the above criteria. However, all publications that we found presumed that the participants were able to stand for long periods and could carry out co-ordinated sequences of movement with no difficulty. There was not one publication which we could fully recommend that described a set of exercises which would be safe and appropriate for people with MS. Most publications do presume, naturally enough, that the readers have no difficulty with normal standing, sitting and walking and can co-ordinate movements in a fluid manner.

We therefore developed our own set of training materials that included written information sheets, a video and an audiotape. This book contains the original instructions and is further enriched by some additional material on cultivating a sense of safety as well as additional material on strategies to cope with stress and trauma.

Results of the research study

I feel I have improved because of finding a form of exercise that does not cause pain or fatigue and finding a peace within myself.
(Comment from participant in the research study)

We asked everyone in the study to rate whether the following problems had improved by the end of the research study. These results were compared with a control group of people who had MS, but who did not engage in the qigong.

Who were the participants?

We recruited people with MS through local physiotherapists and general practitioners. All the people in the study had a diagnosis of secondary progressive MS, which had been given by a consultant neurologist. To be accepted into the study people had to fulfil the following criteria:

1. They had to be able to make their own way to the hospital.

2. They had to be capable of understanding written and verbal instructions.

3. They had to be able to manipulate a pencil sufficiently in order to fill in questionnaires.

4. They had to be prepared to make a commitment to regular practice.

These criteria, of course, ruled out people who would have a very high degree of physical or cognitive impairment. Participants had, however, to be experiencing at least one symptom that severely affected their life on an ongoing basis.

Table 2.1 Results of the research study investigating improvements after a course of qigong

	Percentage of qigong participants who improved	Percentage of control group participants who improved
Walking distance	50	0
Walking steadiness	37.5	0
Ability to stand	37.5	0
Balance	25	0
Tremor	12.5	0
Spasms	25	12.5
Bladder problems	50	12.5
Stiffness in joints	62.5	0
General well-being	62.5	25
Fatigue	37.5	12.5
Depression	12.5	12.5
Anxiety	12.5	12.5
Concentration	25	0
Numbness in fingers or feet	37.5	0
Fine motor control	25	0
Ability to move legs	37.5	12.5
Co-ordination	25	12.5
Sleep	12.5	12.5
Constipation	37.5	25
Pain	37.5	0

In order to obtain research funding and to meet the concerns of the Hospital Research and Ethics Committee, we had to compare our results from the qigong programme with a control group. Comparison with a control group is particularly important for studies concerning MS, as the symptoms of MS vary a lot, so it could be that any supposed treatment was actually just measuring a natural variation of symptoms that would have happened anyway, without any intervention.

Furthermore, just the aspect of being talked to by a researcher and asked how you are feeling, is mildly therapeutic for some people. As you can see, some of the people in the control group did experience a slight improvement in some of their symptoms. However, the qigong group reported improvements on a much bigger scale.

Ideally in a research study large numbers of people are recruited and they are randomly allocated to different groups. However, with the funds available to us we were only able to investigate a fairly small sample. We were, therefore, advised by our statistician to use a procedure called 'matching'. Matching means that for every person who is receiving a treatment there has to be a person in the control group who has a similar level of severity in terms of their symptoms.

It wouldn't be of any use to randomly allocate people to a qigong group and to a control group, in order to find that people in the qigong group were performing already at a much higher level than the people in the control group, even before the qigong was carried out. Therefore, every person allocated to the qigong group was matched to someone allocated to the control group in terms of their range and severity of symptoms. Full details of this procedure and the subsequent statistical analysis are available in the scientific articles that were subsequently published in medical journals (Mills, Allen and Carey-Morgan 2000; Mills and Allen 2000). We were also advised that in addition to the person themselves rating any changes, we should also ask a relative or a friend of each participant to rate whether they had also observed any improvement or deterioration.

The results in Table 2.2 show how the two groups compared three months after the programme had finished (Mills and Allen 2000).

Table 2.2 Summary of symptom change at three-month follow-up as rated by qigong participants compared with the control group

	Total no. of symptoms reported	Percentage improvement	Percentage deterioration	Percentage no change
Qigong	114	41	4	55
Control group	118	9	27	64
Qigong relatives' ratings	119	32	8	60

To put Table 2.2 into words, the people who practised qigong reported an improvement in 41 per cent of their symptoms.

This compares to 9 per cent of the control group. Furthermore, only 4 per cent of the qigong group reported any deterioration in their symptoms compared with 27 per cent of the control group.

As well as asking people to keep a check on their symptoms, we also included a more objective measure of balance.

We looked at the established research literature to see how balance has been measured in other studies and were surprised to find there was a delightfully simple test that involved no expense at all. The test, recommended by consultant neurologists, is to note the number of seconds that balance can be maintained whilst standing on one leg.

We carried out this test both before and after the qigong treatment. We also measured it again at the follow-up three months after the end of the study. The results are produced below.

Table 2.3 Number of seconds each qigong
participant could balance on one leg

Participant no.	Pre-qigong	Post-qigong	Follow-up
1	5	10	7
2	5	10	20
3	5	10	7
4	15	40	32
5	5	10	Not given
6	3	3	Dropped out
7	2	4	10
8	5	8	3
Average	5.63	11.88	13.17

What Table 2.3 shows is that nearly all of the participants who took part in the qigong programme managed to almost double the amount of time they could stand on one leg. This improvement in balance was taken over into walking so that approximately 50 per cent of the participants found that they could walk further and walk more steadily than they had been able to prior to the qigong programme.

This improvement in balance through practising qigong had been noted in a previous research study, which had looked at how the principles of tai chi might help elderly people to improve their balance, and so reduce the number of falls they had. We found two studies reported in medical research journals, one by Jacobson *et al.* (1997) and one by Wolf *et al.* (1997); both studies showed that elderly people improved their balance after practising a course of tai chi. The improvement of balance for people with MS is very important. As noted previously, people with MS are very prone to falling over and incurring serious injury from the fall. This has been documented in a recent study by Peterson *et al.* (2008) who found that 50 per cent of a large sample of people with MS reported injurious falls. Therefore, any approach which can improve the ability to balance is very important for people with MS.

The results from our research study were of sufficient magnitude to be taken note of by the UK's National Institute of Clinical Excellence (NICE). The research publication by Mills and Allen (2000) is now cited in the supporting information for UK guidelines on the treatment of MS.

Unfortunately, despite the promising nature of our initial research results there have been no further attempts to mount a larger research study to test out the programme on a larger group.

Research funding in the Western world is largely provided by drug companies and in the case of qigong, there is no drug to be marketed and therefore no profit to be made. One of the hopes of publishing this book is that the potential of qigong in helping to improve the quality of life of people suffering from MS, can be more widely known and may lead to other researchers to apply for funding for more substantial research to be undertaken.

So what did we do?

The actual contents of the programme that we carried out are described fully in Chapters 5 and 6. The tuition was delivered in one-to-one sessions with either Simon Carey-Morgan or Nigel Mills. Sessions were held weekly or fortnightly. Six individual sessions were provided altogether.

In addition to each individual teaching session, every participant was expected to carry out a daily homework practice of at least 30 minutes. Furthermore, each participant was supplied with a video tape of the exercises, an audio tape of the meditation and breathing instructions, and a printed handout.

Thus every participant had an intensive exposure to the programme for a total period of approximately three months on a daily basis.

In order to understand the rationale for the exercises that are found in the main body of this programme I need first of all to go into a little background about the assumptions underlying qigong in terms of 'energy' or 'qi' or 'chi', as it is sometimes called. This is the focus for the following chapter.

Chapter 3

MULTIPLE SCLEROSIS FROM A CHI POINT OF VIEW

What is chi?

Chi's most basic translation refers to the idea of 'energy'. In the West we tend to use the word energy to refer to the obvious fuel sources of oil and coal, or the energy we are increasingly producing from wind power and solar power. However, if we think how the word energy is used in physics we have a much broader use of the term. It is a fundamental proposition in physics that energy and matter are one and the same thing. It is only the speed of vibration, which makes some forms of energy appear solid and other forms of energy to be more like a heat or light, or even radio waves or mobile phone messages.

A good example is the process of combustion. When you look at a piece of wood it looks very solid. There does not seem to be any of this mysterious energy or 'chi' in a bit of old wood. If you were to cut the wood up, or even make it into wood shavings you still would not discover anything that looks much like 'energy'. However, if you were to set light to it, then, hey presto, magic happens, chi appears in the form of heat and light. The speed of vibration of the piece of wood has changed, and what previously appeared solid is now light and heat.

As Einstein described:

E (energy) = M (mass) multiplied by C (speed) squared

It is this more recent conceptualization of energy that the ancient Chinese also described many thousands of years ago. The link between ancient Chinese philosophy and modern physics has been well described in several texts including the classic 'The Tao of Physics' by Capra (1991) and more recently Oschman (2000).

Thus the perception of matter, and that includes our bodies, is dependant on the speed of vibration. We cannot see the energy of mobile phone messages or radiowaves or TV signals because the frequency of vibration is beyond that of visual recognition. However, we can see the more substantial energy format of bones, blood and even nerve fibre because their frequency of vibration is within our visual range.

The Chinese did not just think about this issue philosophically, they also applied it to how they carried out medicine. They saw the human body, not as a collection of tubes and levers, as tends to be the case with Western medicine, but rather an integrated pulsating energy field.

The human body is in a continual amazing process of alchemy. The term alchemy refers to the process whereupon one substance is transformed into another. We take in solid bits of potato, fish, cheese, and lettuce and then within a matter of a few hours this matter is being transformed beyond all recognition and is on its way to becoming blood, bone and nervous tissue. Our school text books in biology describe this change as a chemical process of enzymes actively at work. However, behind every chemical change there is an energy change and accompanying changes in the surrounding energy fields.

The ancient Chinese also observed that energy (or chi) fields do not operate in isolation but are affected by other energy fields.

In the West we refer to one aspect of this phenomenon as gravity. We acknowledge that the movement of the moon causes changes, which results in the tide-like movements of the oceans.

We also acknowledge that the energy field of a mobile phone is sufficient enough to disrupt the functioning of aircraft or medical equipment. We are therefore asked to turn off our mobile phones when in hospital or aeroplane environments.

Strangely, whilst we recognize that the energy field of the oceans is affected by the energy field of the moon and we accept that the energy field of sensitive equipment can be affected by the energy field of mobile phones, there is considerably more resistance to an acceptance that the far more sensitive energy field of the human nervous system may be positively and negatively affected by surrounding energy fields.

Are you likely to feel better, in yourself, if you were to walk through a forest on a spring day or to walk through an office building full computers and mobile phones and microwave cookers?

Chapter 4 describes some of the arguments for how mobile phones and WiFi may adversely affect our health. Now and again there is a newspaper headline concerning this connection, but we all carry on as usual. There are massive personal and commercial interests at work to blind us to this.

Ancient Chinese medicine did not have to contend with the possible adverse effects of mobile phones. It concerned itself more with the potentially positive, beneficial effects that can be gained from the energy field of the surrounding universe. This is poetically stated in an ancient Chinese text (Hua-Ching 1993) as: 'Make love with the invisible subtle origin of the universe, and you will give yourself everything you need.'

In our Western culture we tend to think of ourselves as isolated bits of machinery that rush around, occasionally bumping into other bits of machinery in order to make further bits of machinery. Our view of ourselves is currently still informed by the developments of the industrial revolution and surrounding ourselves with cars and mechanical gadgets.

The world of the ancient Chinese is informed by being immersed in nature and drawing inspiration from the seasons and the patterns of the weather. Maybe, as more recent notions of modern physics become more widely accepted and as we become more immersed in virtual reality and electronic versions of reality, our conceptualization of ourselves will also shift away from one of 'levers and tubes' to something different. Unfortunately our conceptualisation will probably still be removed from the intimate observation of nature, as described by the ancient Chinese.

At this point we can attempt to explore the disorder of multiple sclerosis (MS) with a new point of view of energy or 'chi'.

Multiple sclerosis as disturbed 'chi'

The basic premise of this program is that the symptoms of MS are a reflection of an underlying disturbance in the energy flows of the body. If the energy flows of the body can be brought into harmony, the improved bioelectric template of the body will give rise to the necessary biochemical changes that need to take place.

Thus the order of change that needs to occur, according to Chinese medicine, is that first the energy system of the body has to be bought into a healthy pattern; the necessary biochemical changes then automatically follow to induce health in the blood, tissues and nervous system of the body.

Attempting to heal the body through making interventions to biochemistry is to Chinese medicine rather like trying to fix a car which is miss-firing by adding additives to the petrol, when it is really the electronic timing mechanism of the car which is at fault.

So what would a harmonized energy field look like? There are different levels of answer to this question. Chinese medicine provides a detailed description of the energy circuitry of the body. The 'wiring' which carries the chi throughout the body is called the 'meridian' system. The energy channels can become blocked or distorted and ill health then follows. It is these energy channels or meridians on which acupuncture is used to stimulate or quieten the body's flow of energy. In Chinese medicine there is a complex 'technology' of how the meridians affect each other and how the meridians can be unblocked, stimulated or quietened to help recovery from certain disorders. A detailed explanation of this technology is far beyond the scope of this book. The interested reader is referred to texts by Kaptchuk (2000) and Beinfield and Korngold (1991) for full explanations of the energy system that underpins Chinese medicine.

People with MS suffer from a large variety of different symptoms. Symptoms may include spasticity of muscles, loss of sensation, incontinence, loss of balance, fatigue and memory problems. The usual medical explanation given for such a variety of symptoms is that there has been a destruction of the myelin sheath. The myelin sheath is the insulation around the nerve fibres.

If you were to think of a conventional piece of wire as an inner strand of copper which carries the electricity with an insulating plastic sheet around it, then the plastic insulating sheath is the electrical parallel of the myelin sheath around a nerve fibre. If the plastic insulating sheath was to deteriorate after a while, the electric current running along the wire would short and jump across to other wires, or would try and find the quickest path to earth through the surrounding metal work.

Imagine for a moment the insides of a computer with masses of wiring. Imagine the insulation around some of that wiring started to deteriorate and so sparks of electricity started to jump to other wires and to the metal casing. Would the computer continue to function normally? No. Imagine now the even greater complexity of the human nervous system and the problems that are likely to result if nerve fibres start getting their messages mixed up. This is MS.

Why does the myelin sheath break down?

The medical evidence suggests that the breakdown of the myelin sheath is caused by the immune system going haywire and attacking the healthy tissue of the myelin sheath. This causes inflammation and ultimate destruction. This phenomenon is usually described in biochemical terms and changes in immune functioning.

However recent advances in the field of psychoneuroimmunology indicate that the immune system does not act in isolation but is a part of a complex pattern of interaction between psychological appraisal, nervous system reaction and endocrine functioning.

> The sympathetic nervous system extends into all parts of the body involved in the immune response, including the thymus, the bone marrow, the spleen, lymph nodes and Peyer's patches. (Waksman 1994)

Thus changes in nervous arousal and stress responses also trigger biochemical changes in the immune system.

It is the functioning of the nervous system and its vulnerability to the manipulations of subtle energy which are the focus of the ancient Chinese medicine. For a disease process to be initiated in the human body an ancient Chinese medical model would say that there must first of all be a disturbance in the subtle energy patterns in or around the body.

The medicine of ancient China promoted efforts of keeping the subtle energy patterns in a healthier form so as to prevent the onset of disease. Ancient Chinese physicians were only paid by the patients whilst the patients kept well. The development of disease in a patient meant that the physician had not been doing his job and so the payment would then stop.

The physician therefore focused on using preventative approaches to medicine. This included dietary advice, the use of herbs and acupuncture and the practice of qigong. Qigong is essentially a method of harmonizing and keeping healthy the subtle energy patterns in the body so that disease does not develop. This was poetically described by Su Wen (quoted in Jahnke 2002) as follows:

> To wait for the illness to develop before remedying it,
> for the disorder to form,
> before taking care of it,
> is to wait until one is thirsty before digging a well,
> to wait for the battle,
> before forging the weapons.
> Is this not too late?

Note how this contrasts to Western medicine, where the approach tends to be to wait until the illness is full-blown before treatment commences.

MINIMIZING NEGATIVE INFLUENCES ON YOUR NERVOUS SYSTEM

Western medicine has been unable to identify one single external factor that may precipitate multiple sclerosis (MS). There are many theories of possible factors, which increase a person's vulnerability to MS. These factors include exposure to viruses, stress, Western style diet and exposure to certain forms of electromagnetic or microwave radiation. At first sight, these factors appear to be very diverse and have no link between them. However, when we take a 'chi' perspective, what they do all have in common is that they all affect the body's pattern of subtle energy. Each of the above factors affects the way in which the body is able to transmit electrochemical information through the nervous system.

We may use the analogy again of a very sensitive piece of electrical equipment, such as is used in heart rate monitors or navigation equipment on an airplane. If you were to expose that sensitive equipment to other electromagnetic fields or if the equipment was not maintained or if it was exposed to some form of toxic chemicals, then that machinery would malfunction. In order to help it function properly again one would have to first minimize the exposure of the machinery to the adverse outside influences.

There would be little point in tinkering with the flow of the frequency and quantity of electricity through your delicate instrument, if you had not beforehand removed or minimized the outside negative influences. So, it is similar with a 'chi' approach to the treatment of health problems. Before embarking on the treatment programme one needs to consider whether there may be factors in the environment which could be having a negative effect on the flow of subtle energy through your body. That is the focus of this chapter.

We will look at three main influences that may have an adverse effect on your nervous system:

- Stress.

- Electromagnetic fields and microwave radiation.

- Nutrition.

- Fluid intake.

Stress

It is now well acknowledged that MS can be made worse by stress. A study reported in the *British Medical Journal* (Buljevac *et al.* 2003) reported that the experience of traumatic life events was associated with double the risk of an exacerbation of MS. The authors describe how other studies have also shown that stress has an adverse effect on the immune system. More recently a study from Israel has shown that exacerbations of MS were over three times more likely in the 2006, 33-day war, compared with the pre-war period (Golan, Somer and Dishon 2008).

Our response to stress is governed by a basic biological mechanism called the 'fight–flight–freezing mechanism'. When we sense that we under stress our biology initially prepares us for action, to either fight the stressor or flee from it, or sometimes to 'freeze'. In the first two instances the sympathetic nervous system becomes activated, the heart rate is increased, adrenaline is secreted, blood flow increases. In recent years it has also been found that the immune system is involved in this preparation for action:

> Nerve fibers of the sympathetic nervous system extend into all parts of the body involved in the immune response, including the thymus, the bone marrow, the spleen, lymph nodes and Peyer's patches. (Waksman 1994)

We know that MS is affected by the immune system; we also know that stress and trauma affect the immune system. It is therefore not a great leap to suggest that stress may well affect MS.

The interesting and rather disturbing thing about trauma is that it is not only distressing when you experience a traumatic event, but it is also disturbing when you cast your mind back to it and think about it again. The nervous system is then affected all over again.

You have probably noticed that when the memory of a previous traumatic event is triggered you may have experienced a wave of distressing thoughts and feelings. This can sometimes be accompanied by very real, and sometimes frightening, physical sensations.

What is happening here? Bringing to mind the memory of the trauma has activated your sympathetic nervous system. It is as though your nervous system thinks the threat of the trauma is still present. Your nervous system is, in effect, preparing you for action against a threat, which is no longer there.

For some people this preparation involves being on 'red alert', expecting danger from all directions; this is known as 'hyperarousal'.

For other people their system seems to go into 'shut down' or 'hypoarousal' (freezing).

It is useful to think about this process with reference to what happens in animals. Some animals respond to danger by fighting or fleeing; this requires that their sympathetic nervous system becomes activated so the heart can pump faster and the muscles can work better. Other animals respond to danger with 'freezing'. The advantage of freezing is that you look as if you are dead, so any predator that is passing by isn't interested in eating you.

A further use of this strategy has been suggested (Levine 1997): if you are going to be eaten or destroyed in some way then the pain of your final moments will be numbed by this complete shut down and closing off from sensation.

As humans faced with danger, we resort to the same basic mechanisms of fight, flight or freezing. However in humans, more than animals, the mechanism seems to get 'stuck', so even if the danger has passed we are often left in a state of either hyperarousal or hypoaraousal.

Whilst part of you knows, rationally, that the threat is no longer there, another part of you is convinced that you are in danger, and needs to keep your protective mechanism going.

Scientists have even identified the two parts of the brain that react in these two different ways: the outer layer of the brain, known as the cortex, is the part that makes sense of things rationally, whilst it is the lower part of the brain, known as the limbic system, which reacts in a more primitive way. However much you try telling yourself that there is nothing to be frightened of, the limbic system just doesn't seem to hear and carries on pumping out the chemicals, which make you feel anxious.

In terms of the effect this has on MS, it has been shown, as mentioned previously, that when the nervous system is responding to stress, the immune system is also affected, which in turn is likely to affect the progress of autoimmune disorders, such as MS.

It is therefore likely to be useful to learn to react to stress (whether real or imagined) in a way which does not activate your sympathetic nervous system and in a way which does not have an adverse effect on your vulnerability to MS. Qigong is not just a physical exercise system, it is also a way of cultivating a state of mind which is calmer and more able to cope with stress. The exercises presented in Chapters 5, 6 and 7 are particularly useful for re-training the way your body and mind react to stress.

Electromagnetic fields and microwave radiation

We have never before in all of human history subjected the human body to such a mass of electromagnetic stimulation or surrounded ourselves with such a web of microwave radiation. We have also in all of human history never before seen such a rise in disorders such as MS, chronic fatigue, and Parkinson's disease. Whilst modern medicine makes great strides in coming up with ways of fighting bacteria and viruses and removing malfunctioning pieces of anatomy, it remains at something of a loss to know what to do in these more diffuse systemic malfunctions of the human system.

This is maybe because the cause of these more diffuse problems cannot be traced to one single bacterium, one single virus, or one single malfunction in anatomy or circulation. Disorders such as MS concern the whole system in a rather diffuse network fashion. So it is with the effects of electromagnetic and microwave radiation, the whole system is being affected in a diffuse network manner.

If electromagnetic and microwave radiation could be seen, we would be seeing ourselves as continuously bombarded. If we saw ourselves not as discrete entities which end at the boundary of our skin, but rather as modern physics tells us, fluctuating subtle electric fields, then we would perhaps have a better appreciation of how the microwave radiation coming from a mobile phone is bound to affect the ebb and flow of our own fluctuating subtle flow of energy. Recent research from the University of Lund in Sweden (Salford *et al.* 2003; Nittby 2008) has shown that the permeability of the blood–brain barrier in rats is increased after exposure to mobile phone radiation. The studies have also found neuronal damage several weeks after exposure to mobile phone radiation.

It is not possible to remove ourselves from the radiation all around us. Many people would find it impossible to function in today's culture without the use of a mobile phone, computer, microwave oven, etc. There are however some practical steps you can take to protect the delicate subtle energy circuitry of your own system and minimize your exposure to the influences of radiation and electric fields around you. Four of the most important steps you can take are identified below:

Mobile phones

If you want to give yourself the best possible chance of recovery, only use a conventional landline. If you must use a mobile phone, do not place it next to your ear until the phone is connected with the other person you wish to speak to. Hold the phone as far away from your ear as you can whilst still being able to hear the other person. Check the SAR rating of your phone. This should be listed in the information given with your phone or on the website of the manufacturer. An SAR rating indicates how much radiation is coming from your phone. If you must use a mobile phone, choose one with the lowest SAR rating available.

Computers

A wireless connection for your computer means that you are bathing your house in a constant flow of electrical energy, the consequences of which are currently unclear. Professor Challis, chairman of the UK government's Mobile Telecommunications and Health Research Group has recommended that children should not sit with a laptop on their lap, as they are then being exposed to a similar level of radiation as that from a mobile phone (Fleming 2007). The Austrian Medical Association is recommending a ban on WiFi use in schools. Dr Oberfeld, head of Environmental Health and Medicine in Salzburg, has described WiFi as 'dangerous to sensitive people'.

If you wish to give yourself the best possible chance of recovery consider changing to a cable broadband connection. If you are totally addicted to WiFi, and can't imagine life without it, then make sure your computer is turned off when you are not using it, otherwise you are unnecessarily exposing your nervous system to WiFi radiation. Particularly ensure the WiFi is not active at night and therefore not bathing you in further radiation when asleep. Turn off your computer when not in use.

Placement of bed

Make sure your bed is not in the very near vicinity of electrical equipment such as alarm clocks or mobile phone chargers or electric cabling which has an active electric current.

Microwave ovens

The debate about the safety of microwave ovens continues (see www.cancersalves.com/articles/microwave). Some authorities argue that microwave radiation changes the biochemical structure of the food, so that it becomes harmful to human health. Many people with MS use microwave cookers as they appear to be easier to use than conventional methods of cooking. You may like to do a search on the issues involved and decide for yourself!

Nutrition

The topic of nutrition is massive. There have been many books and articles about the possible level of nutrition in MS (see Buckley 2007 and Jelinek 2005 for recent reviews and some practical guidelines). It is beyond the scope of this book to review all this information here. In terms of one of the main themes of this book, which is trying to encourage a lowering of arousal of the sympathetic nervous system, then there are particular issues with respect to nutrition. If MS is aggravated by stress and anything which has an adverse effect on the nervous system, then one may be well advised to avoid foods that over-stimulate the nervous system and mimic the effects of stress.

The aspects of nutrition that particularly affect the nervous system are those foods which contain caffeine. These include coffee, tea, chocolate and cola, which tend to result in activation of the sympathetic nervous system. As mentioned previously, the discipline of psychoneuroimmunology has well demonstrated that activation of the sympathetic nervous system also has adverse effects on the immune system. Since MS is essentially a disorder of the immune system you may find it useful to avoid foods which affect the immune system.

There are many other dietary recommendations for people with MS including the recommendation to take omega 3 supplements; to eat five portions of fruit and vegetables; increase vitamin D intake and to reduce saturated fat intake and avoid allergens. The interested reader is recommended to listen to your medical advisor, read the texts by Buckley (2007) and Jelinek (2005) and then make your own decision!

The whole aspect of how nutrition affects the body from a Chinese medicine point of view is dealt with very clearly in an interesting book by Leggett (1999).

Fluid intake

People with MS sometimes have bladder difficulties and in order to minimize the number of occasions on which they have to rush to the toilet they may try and reduce their fluid intake.

However, water makes up 60–70 per cent of men's body weight; women have 55–65 per cent because of their higher body fat content and babies have an even higher water content of 75 per cent.

In terms of the relationship between chi and fluid it can be useful to think of the analogy of a car battery. There is no point in trying to charge up a car battery which is empty of fluid. The charge just won't hold!

A fluid deficiency of just 2 per cent of your body weight is sufficient to start reducing your ability to concentrate and carry out everyday tasks. Approximately two litres of fluid intake per day is needed as the body eliminates this quantity of fluid every day through the skin, lungs, bladder and intestines.

If you have insufficient water intake your blood plasma and total blood volume decrease. The reduced blood flow to the heart results in the body becoming poorly supplied with blood and oxygen. If deprived of water, the brain, blood, muscles and other organs cannot function properly. In addition to concentration problems you are also likely to feel tired and suffer with long-term constipation and circulatory problems.

However don't drink too much either! The analogy of the car battery continues to hold good, in terms of overdrinking. If you kept on pouring water into your car battery, the electrolytes would be over-diluted and the electric charge would not be able to build up sufficiently. So providing just the right amount of fluid is important. One and a half to two litres of fluid a day is a good target.

Chapter 5

QIGONG EXERCISES: CREATING INNER SPACE, RELEASING TENSION AND DISCOVERING ALIGNMENT

The programme is divided into seven stages. In this chapter we will look at stages 1 to 4. In the next chapter we will look at stages 5 to 7.

The stages:

1. Cultivating safety.

2. Releasing tension – stretching, shaking and bouncing.

3. Encouraging alignment – the standing and sitting postures.

4. Self-healing – creating inner space.

5. Developing a sense of balance.

6. Finding your feet again.

7. Meditation – gathering and centring.

When to practise?

Practise first thing in the morning, before breakfast, and last thing in the evening, before bed.

The morning session

The reason for the morning session is to shake off the constrictions of the night and to set up an energetic template, which can act as a healthy starting point for the day ahead. It is much harder to settle into qigong once your mind has become busy and you are rushing about on your 'to do' list. Furthermore, first thing in the morning is good because your energy will flow easier when you haven't eaten, your mind is stiller, the surrounding environment is stiller, and also, traditionally, the 'chi' of the earth is at its greatest in the morning. The traditional qigong guidance is to practise between 5 am and 7 am. If that thought fills you with horror, just make it as early as you can! Once you feel comfortable and safe doing the exercises you may like to do a shorter version of stage 1, about cultivating a feeling of safety. However, initially, it is useful to try out all the different ways of cultivating safety and then choose to focus on the one or two, which you find particularly beneficial.

As mentioned at the end of Chapter 4, we generally wake up somewhat dehydrated; it is therefore a good idea to drink at least two mugs of warm herbal tea or warm water with lemon, throughout your morning session. This flushes your system of residual toxins, and provides a better fluid base from which to absorb the chi. Remember the advice at the end of Chapter 4: there is no point in trying to charge up a car battery which is empty of fluid. The charge just won't hold!

The evening session

The reason for the evening session is to calm down at the end of the day and set up an energetic template for a restful night's sleep. If you enter sleep with your mind buzzing with TV, or conversations just had on the telephone, or books just read, then your mind and your nervous system and your body, continues trying to process that information. Nighttime can be a very important time for healing. But as I have said several times already and will probably say several more times before the end of this book: healing requires spaciousness. Doing a 'just before bed' qigong session is an excellent way to calm down from the stresses of the day, bring your nervous system back into balance and set up a spacious energetic template for a night of self-healing. For the evening session it is good to start with stage 1, the safe place exercise, and then move on to stage 3. Many people, myself included, find that stage 2, releasing tension through the stretches, is too energizing, and so then find it harder to get to sleep. I would therefore recommend leaving out the stretching and shaking for the evening practice.

What is important, for the follower of this programme, is how it is possible through your own efforts, to release the blocks in your own system and bring the energy flow of your body into harmony. This process will only be fully successful if it is followed in a certain order.

Stage 1: Cultivating safety

If you have multiple sclerosis (MS) or any other neurological condition, you probably feel very vulnerable in your body. The process of moving and balancing that you once took for granted, is no longer so certain. Even just thinking about the fact that you have MS may trigger a sense of anxiety. This anxiety and sense of vulnerability is accompanied by physiological changes. Your sympathetic nervous system becomes activated, the heart beats slightly faster, the blood pressure increases, the muscles constrict; it as though you are preparing to fight or flee or for some people to freeze. This arousal of the sympathetic nervous system is not conducive to healing and it is not conducive to learning a new skill especially not a new skill like qigong, which requires a sense of calm attention.

It is therefore useful to spend a few minutes, particularly at the end of the day, cultivating a sense of safety. If you enter into this exercise programme in a state of fear, then there will be no spaciousness inside you, only tightness and constriction. For the healing process to be helped, spaciousness is required, and spaciousness requires a sense of safety.

How to experience safety in the body

If you have a tendency to anxiety and panic, you are probably holding tension in the upper part of your body around the head and around the upper chest. You may also have a tendency to restrict your breathing. The breath becomes shallow and rapid, the shoulders often become tight and the neck also becomes tight; a sense of tension in the head often accumulates.

To allow a safer feeling to fill your body, it can be good to allow that tension to move and go down towards the floor and into the ground. Finding a pathway for the hyperarousal of the head and chest to flow to the ground can be a vitally important discovery.

EXERCISE 1: SOFTENING AND LETTING GO

Sit in a straight-backed chair, have both feet flat on the ground. Don't crumple into the chair, but allow your back to be long and your belly to be soft. Have the sense that you are allowing your weight to go down into the chair and through the chair into the ground. It is important that your legs are uncrossed and your feet are flat on the floor. Sense the ground underneath your feet.

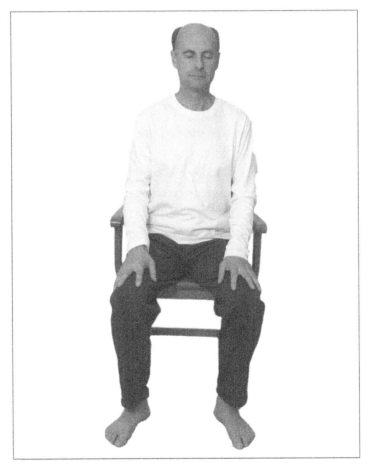

Sitting posture

Now, tune into the sensations in your body that you notice at the present time.

Start at your head and work your way down, centimetre by centimetre.

Any sensations of tension, tightness or agitation can be given space and allowed to flow down through the body until the tension melts away into the floor.

What do you notice across the top of your head? Breathe in to the top of your head. Let it soften, let it go, follow it down to your feet and out into the floor.

What do you notice across your forehead? As you breathe in notice your forehead, as you breathe out, let it soften, let it go, allow the tension to flow, down to your feet and out into the floor.

What do you notice around your jaw? As you breathe in, bring your attention to your jaw. As you breathe out, let it soften, let it go, let the sensations go down to your feet and out into the floor.

What do you notice around your neck? Let it soften, let it go, follow it down to your feet and out into the floor.

What do you notice across your shoulders? Let it soften, let it go, follow it down to your feet and out into the floor.

What do you notice across your chest? Let it soften, let it go, follow it down to your feet.

What do you notice in your upper arms? Let it soften, let it go, follow it down to your fingertips and out into the air.

What do you notice in your elbows? Let it soften, let it go, follow it down to your fingertips and out into the air.

What do you notice in your forearms and wrists? Let it soften, let it go, follow it down to your fingertips and out into the air.

What do you notice in your hands? Let it soften, let it go, follow it down to your fingertips and out into the air.

What do you notice down the length of your back? Let it soften, let it go, follow it down to your feet and out into the floor.

What do you notice in your belly? Let it soften, let it go, follow it down to your feet and out into the floor.

What do you notice in your hips and pelvic area? Let it soften, let it go, follow it down to your feet and out into the floor.

What do you notice in your thighs? Let it soften, let it go, follow it down to your feet and out into the floor.

What do you notice in your knees? Let it soften, let it go, follow it down to your feet and out into the floor.

What do you notice in your calves? Let it soften, let it go, follow it down to your feet and out into the floor.

What do you notice in your ankles and feet? Let it soften, let it go, follow it down to your toes and out into the floor.

This simple technique by itself can often be of considerable help in encouraging a sense of safety in the body.

The way in which this exercise is taught is subtly, but very importantly, different from 'just relaxation'. Relaxation exercises are often used as a distraction from your experience, somewhere else to place your attention instead of on the distressing experience. Here the emphasis is not on distracting yourself from the distress, but rather *allowing* the distress to flow down through your body, so that it is no longer held in one place. So, in effect you are giving yourself an empowering experience of 'surviving' your emotions rather than distracting yourself.

Grounding

The process of bringing your attention down to the ground is sometimes called 'grounding'. It can be helped by placing your attention below your feet, and imagining your awareness being drawn to the very centre of the earth and the centre of safety.

Sometimes it is useful to use the analogy of the roots of a tree, as described in the exercise below.

EXERCISE 2: GROUNDING

Imagine your awareness searching down, between the rocks. Just as tree roots search for moisture and nutrients so your awareness can search for connection to the earth.

Seek out the grounding influence of the planet beneath your feet.

Sense the molten core at the centre of the earth, let yourself be open to the magnetic pull of the magnetic core.

Imagine yourself to be like a collection of iron filings; allow the magnetic core of the earth to bring all your scattered 'charge' into a more unified pattern.

Feel how you have a tendency to be drawn to the centre of the earth.

(See Appendix at the end of the book for an expanded version of this exercise.)

This connection with the earth can also be encouraged through activities which remind us of our dependence on the earth such as gardening or walking in the countryside.

To cultivate a feeling of safety and shift your nervous system into 'safe mode' it is good to practise this cultivation of connection with the earth on a daily basis; do not leave it until you are feeling anxious. The practice and skill need to be cultivated when you are feeling fairly calm and in a non-threatening environment. When you have developed some skill in increasing your connection with the earth, then it is useful to test it out in an anxiety provoking situation. The task then is to allow the waves of anxiety to travel through the body and to pass into the earth, to allow the earth to soak up the anxiety.

Cultivating safety through breathing

To release anxiety – breathe out! It is amazing how many people hold on to their breath when they are anxious. The anxiety then stays in the body, and the whole situation escalates. Alternatively some people begin to breathe in short sharp breaths; this is known as hyperventilation, and also triggers further anxiety.

If a full out-breath has been achieved then the in-breath will follow naturally. This avoids a tendency to suck air in or to pull air in forcibly, which can in itself create a heightened state of tension and anxiety. Allowing a full out-breath can encourage a general sense of letting go and releasing.

In qigong there is also a recommendation to allow the abdomen to expand on the in-breath and fall back on the out-breath.

EXERCISE 3: BREATHING

Adopt the same sitting posture as in Exercise 1.
Feet flat on the ground.
Spine long.
Belly soft.
Notice how you are breathing at the moment.
Notice if there are any parts of the breathing process which seem to be tight or 'held'.
Bring your attention to those areas.

Give permission for those areas to soften.

Notice if the breath deepens.

Allow the belly to become part of the breath.

Allow the belly to expand on the in-breath.

Allow the belly to fall back on the out-breath.

When you feel you have allowed your belly to become part of the breath, you can also experiment with seeing if you can allow the lower back to expand on the in-breath and fall back on the out-breath.

In addition to increased oxygenation of the blood and the brain and calming of the autonomic nervous system, this relaxed abdominal breathing also has the effect of anchoring your awareness more fully into the body and away from the 'chatter' of the mind.

It should be noted here that some schools of qigong teach a 'forced breathing' technique. It is my experience that this can sometimes be counterproductive for people suffering with anxiety as it sets up a situation where one part of the body is trying to do one thing and another is trying to do something else. So for the purpose of cultivating a bodily sense of safety, I generally use words such as 'allowing' or 'giving permission to' or 'softening'. If this attitude of allowing and softening can be cultivated then the body will find its own fuller way of breathing without any battle having to be entered into.

Opening to allow safety and nourishment to be 'received': the light stream exercise

In addition to safety being cultivated from within, some people also find it useful to allow a safe feeling to come into their body from outside. This is sometimes called qi from heaven or 'the light stream' exercise.

EXERCISE 4: THE LIGHT STREAM

Adopt the same sitting posture as in the previous exercises.

Ask yourself:

'If I was to allow myself to receive a feeling of safety and nourishment, which part of my body would that feeling of safety enter through?'

'If that feeling of safety was to be represented by a coloured light, then what colour would be of most benefit to me right now?'

Allow that possibility, just now, of allowing that particular colour light to enter into that part of your body and allow it to circulate through your body.

How does your posture change, as that feeling of safety and nourishment spreads right through your body and mind?

Allow that coloured light to come right into your very being.

What do you notice?

Inspiration from animals

I mentioned previously that the Chinese took great inspiration from their observation of animals. There are in fact deeper forms of qigong which are inspired by, for example, the monkey, the tiger, the eagle and the turtle. Some of these animals are not very accessible to us as role models unless we frequently visit a zoo. However, we do not have to look really far to find other animal teachers in our environment. Maybe the dog lying on your sofa, or the cat curled up in your laundry basket. Notice how your dog or cat almost merges into the object on which they are sitting. They are not worrying about tomorrow and they are not turning over the events of yesterday, they are just here, just now. It as if they are being re-charged; one can almost imagine that they have plugged themselves in to the re-charging mechanism of the universe, and are absorbing chi all over their body surface. Of course they can rush if they need to, when chasing prey or running away. However, in between times, they make the most of the opportunity to come back to their core and re-charge. If you happen to have access to a tortoise then you can see this process at work even more clearly. Notice the slowness of movement and steadiness of step, no rushing, just taking time to absorb the chi. No wonder tortoises live for over 100 years; they are masters of qigong!

We humans often seem to have lost the ability to switch off, unless asleep. We have lost the ability to go into standby; we find it difficult to enter an 'awake but resting' mode. If there is a gap in our lives, if the to-do list is all done, then we tend to turn on the television, pick up a book, turn on the radio; we seek to stimulate our sympathetic nervous system, we seek the ups and downs of fear that we can gain from the media. We find 'nothing to do' more aversive than the stimulation of fear. In so doing we deprive our body of the opportunity to self-heal.

So, take a seat opposite your resting pet, watch, sense their rhythm of breathing, notice how they manage to switch off, whilst remaining on stand-by. Then see if you can do it too.

Stage 2: Releasing tension – stretching, shaking and bouncing

I have developed a confidence in getting to know my body in a different way. (Comment from participant in the research study)

The ancient Chinese approach to medicine taught the importance of change from one state to another. You cannot stay resting all the time; once you have rested you need to move. If you were to stay resting all the time then your muscles would become flaccid, the heart would become out of condition, the digestive organs would stagnate. The 'Yin' of rest needs to move into the 'Yang' of movement and then back again to Yin. Just as the energy from the sun moves from brightness to dark, so too our activity state needs to move from activity to relaxation and back to activity again.

The dog or cat on your couch will not stay there forever, it will eventually stretch itself out, and go off in search of food or adventure.

Notice how your pet manages the transition from resting to activity...with stretching!

Stretching is a vitally important process and again something that we humans seem to have 'civilized out' of ourselves. We recognize the need for a transition, we recognize that we feel groggy and need to somehow wake up in order to face the tasks of the day. However, instead of stretching we tend to reach for a strong cup of tea or coffee. The caffeine kick starts the sympathetic nervous system into action. The heart rate increases, the blood pressure is increased and then we feel 'normal'. The price of this 'normal feeling' is one of gradual over-stimulation and eventual exhaustion of the adrenal glands, and furthermore over-stimulation of the immune system. This is very relevant to sufferers of MS. As you are no doubt already aware it is the over-activity of the immune system which is the main problem in MS. Therefore, an important part of your qigong programme is to replace the kick start of caffeine with the natural start of stretching.

Stretching need not be painful. Stretching in qigong is not like the rigorous pushing of circuit training or even yoga. Qigong again takes its inspiration from animals.

If you bring to mind the image of a dog as it stretches in the morning, it is not that the dog is forcing itself to stretch, it looks more like there is something inside the dog which is telling it that it needs to stretch in order to create space for energy to flow again. So it is in qigong; if one can allow oneself to let go of the inner holding then one finds that the body will often spontaneously stretch to take up the space, which has been created through the letting go.

In order for this 'natural stretching' to occur there must first of all be an attitude of wanting to bring your awareness into your body. Often when we are sitting around or we are preoccupied with something, it is as though our mind becomes disconnected from our body. It can feel as though our body is somehow a mass of wiring and plumbing which hangs beneath our head. It can feel as if our body has a life of its own and functions independently from 'us'.

One of the main aims of this qigong programme is to give you a sense of ownership of your body. A sense that 'you' inhabit all of your body. A sense that each time you breathe, you reclaim ownership of every cell, ownership of every muscle and ownership of every nerve. Most important is the feeling that you can enjoy that sense of ownership, that you can enjoy the physical feeling of air going into your lungs, of blood flowing into your fingers, of sounds coming into your ears, of the pure physicalness of being alive.

Wherever there is constriction, tightness or holding on, then healing cannot take place. We need to somehow find a way to soften, to let go, to unwind. It is only then that the healing qualities of chi are able to flow through our system and restore the energy field to its required harmony. This can be understood perhaps more readily if we use the analogy of the hosepipe. When a hosepipe has a heavy weight sitting on it, or if it is tied in a knot, then water will not flow through. In this analogy, the water is the chi.

Thus although chi is energetic in its nature it still requires a system which is open enough for it to flow unimpeded. Hence the discipline of yoga advocates sometimes quite vigorous stretching to open up the system sufficiently for that which is known in yoga as 'prana' to be able to flow through the body. In qigong the benefits of stretching are also recognized. However, the stretching is usually less subtle than that of yoga. The aim in qigong is more to let go of the inner holding so that the body stretches itself, almost spontaneously. So, let's start.

EXERCISE 5: STRETCHING

These exercises are best done standing; however if standing is difficult they can also be carried out kneeling or sitting.

Standing version

Shoes off, so that you can feel your contact with the ground.

Feel the contact of your feet with the ground.

Make sure your knees are slightly bent.

Bring your attention to your shoulders.

Roll the shoulders around, both together, going backwards. Make this movement gentle. Try and cultivate the sense that your shoulders can, if you let them, move all by themselves.

Feel how the rest of your body can stay relaxed whilst performing this movement. Do at least five repetitions of this backward movement of the shoulders.

Repeat with the shoulders circling forwards.

When the shoulders come to a rest, you may feel that your head wants to 'shake'. If so let it shake!

Next, notice how the movement of the shoulders can become transmitted to the spine and the back.

Relax your hips and the whole pelvic area. Allow the pelvis to move at the same time as the shoulders are moving. Allow the knees to bend to accommodate the movement. Allow the pelvis to swing backwards and forwards.

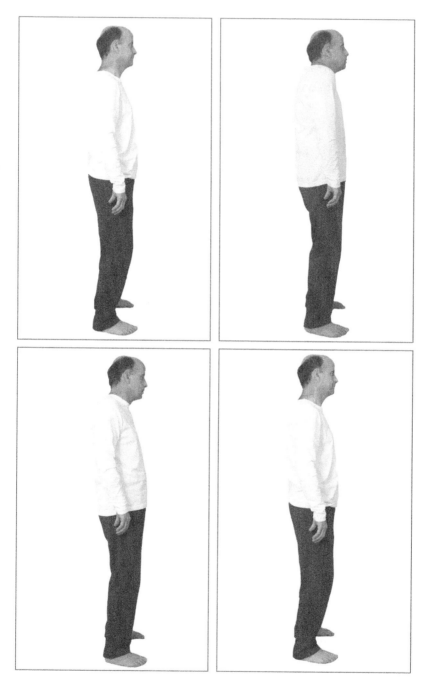

Shoulder circling

Notice how I am using the word 'allowing', not forcing. You should feel as if the pelvis wants to move all by itself not that you are forcing it to move.

Notice the connection between the pelvis and the shoulders. Notice how the spine can undulate following an S type shape as it connects the movement of the shoulders with the movement of the pelvis.

Notice how the movement goes right down into your thighs and the calves.

Notice how the movement of your body involves a shifting of weight from your heels to the balls of the feet.

See if you can relax the muscles of the neck so that the neck and head can also become involved in this undulating movement.

So, after a few minutes the undulating movement is being conveyed through the whole of the body, from the feet right to the top of the head.

You may notice a tendency to yawn or to sigh. Even to cry or to laugh. If so, these are all signs that blocked chi is being released and energy is beginning to flow more freely.

Kneeling version

If you do not feel sufficiently stable standing on your feet then the same benefits can be achieved from a kneeling version of the above exercise. Place a large cushion or other soft material under your knees. If you are able, come into a fairly upright posture so that the thighs are in line with the spine. If this is too difficult for you, then stay kneeling with the thighs against the calves.

As above, commence the movement with the shoulders, then allow the pelvis to also come into play and finally allow the spine to undulate between the movement of the shoulders and the movement of the pelvis.

There are no great 'rights or wrongs' about this exercise. The important thing is to listen to your body, to only do what feels safe for you, given your own ability to keep stable. The main thing you are aiming for, in this exercise, is a loosening of the vertebrae of the spine and the major joints of the shoulders and pelvis.

In qigong, and in Chinese medicine, there are certain areas of the body which are referred to as 'energy gates' (see Bruce Frantzis, *Opening the Energy Gates of Your Body*). Two particularly important areas that act as energy gates are the areas around the shoulders and the pelvis. If these areas become congested or constricted then it is very hard for energy to flow freely through the body. Therefore, this loosening up exercise, which loosens up both the shoulders and the pelvis and the spine in between, is vitally important as a first step in creating some space in the energy channels so that energy can flow again.

Sitting version

If you do not feel comfortable either standing or kneeling, then this exercise can, to some extent, be performed sitting. It is best to use an upright chair such as a kitchen or dining chair. Sit towards the front of the chair so that you are not using the backrest of the chair for support. Once again, start with moving the shoulders. After a few rotations notice how the movement can be transmitted down to the pelvis and notice how the spine can also be brought into the movement so there is a general sense of the body as a whole rising and falling and the spine moving in an S type undulation. Allow the breath to be free, do not force the breath but allow yourself to breathe in and breathe out as the body needs to.

EXERCISE 6: SHAKING

Another excellent way to release blocked chi from the body and mind is through allowing a gentle shaking to take place.

If you feel quite stable on your legs this exercise is best carried out standing. If you are at all concerned about your stability then this exercise should carried out sitting or kneeling.

If you are standing, make sure your knees are slightly bent and your feet are shoulder width apart.

Start with a gentle shaking of the hands and wrists as though trying to shake off water from the finger tips.

Allow the shaking movement to be transmitted up to the elbows and then up to the shoulders.

Keep the shaking gentle. Do not force anything to happen. Your body knows just how much it needs to shake. Listen to your body.

Allow yourself to breathe fully; particularly allow yourself to make full out-breaths. Sighing or yawning increases the ability of this exercise to release congested chi.

Next allow the shaking of the hands and arms to be paralleled by a gentle bouncing of the knees. Make sure the knees stay bent. Next allow the gentle bouncing and shaking movement to be transmitted up to the pelvis.

Feel how, in the words of the famous song, 'The toe bone is connected to the leg bone, the leg bone is connected to the back bone, and the back bone is connected to the head bone and...' etc.

You may at this point find that your body takes on a shaking motion all of its own. This spontaneous form of shaking is an excellent way for the body to release blocked chi and to move towards a state of increased spaciousness and health.

Continue with this shaking and bouncing exercise for as long as you feel comfortable. You should find that the time for which this exercise feels comfortable increases with practice. To start with you may only feel comfortable doing the shaking and bouncing for a minute or two. Then as you gain confidence in your ability to allow the shaking to pass through you, you may find that you continue more of this exercise for five or even ten minutes. Do not over do it. Listen to your body as to when it is the time to stop.

EXERCISE 7: KEEPING YOUR AWARENESS IN THE BELLY

Whilst you are shaking, try to keep the centre of your awareness down in your belly area. In qigong we refer to the 'lower dantien' which is the central area of the body just below the navel. As you breathe in, imagine you are breathing down to this area below the navel. As you breathe out, imagine you are breathing out from this place, just below the navel. Imagine that the central impulse for the shaking and bouncing movement is now coming from this lower dantien area.

Feel the connection between the centre, in the dantien, and the periphery, right out to your finger tips and your toes.

When you feel it is time to stop, take a seat on a kitchen or dining chair with your feet firmly on the ground.

Bring your hands to rest on your lap, one hand cradling the other hand. Imagine that in the cup of your hands you are cradling a small ball. Notice how you can allow your awareness to collect from that ball. As you breath in, it is as though you are breathing into the ball. As you breath out it is as though you are breathing out from the ball. Feel how you can gather your awareness and your energy into this one central place just below the navel.

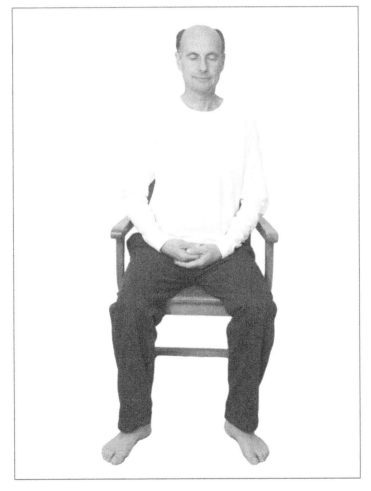

Sitting meditation

The area, called the lower dantien, has a very important role in Chinese medicine and the practice of qigong. This area can act like a reservoir which can collect, absorb and store chi. As you are sitting, allowing your attention to be taken down to the lower dantien, feel how this area can soften, absorb and store the chi which is being released from your previous shaking and bouncing.

Having released some of the tension from your body you are now ready to cultivate more a sense of alignment and of posture, which will encourage the free flow of chi through your body.

Stage 3: Encouraging alignment – the standing and sitting postures

I have an increased awareness of where each part is in relation to each other. (Comment from participant in the research study)

If your body is held in a misaligned way then it is hard for the chi to flow and hard for your awareness to enter your body. It is hard to 'find your feet' if the connection to your feet is blocked. Consider the analogy of water pipes again. If a pipe is kinked then the water will not flow. The exercises below help you to develop a posture which is aligned and which encourages your awareness to enter your body in a fuller way.

EXERCISE 8: STANDING POSTURE

If you have no difficulty standing follow the instructions below. If you have difficulty standing see the sitting version of standing posture.

Standing version

Have your feet shoulder width apart.

Feet should be parallel to each other.

Knees should be soft, i.e. very slightly bent.

Find a way of allowing your weight to go through the centre of your knees into the centre of your feet.

Experiment with shifting your weight, notice the difference in feeling of stability when your weight goes through the back or front of your knees and though the

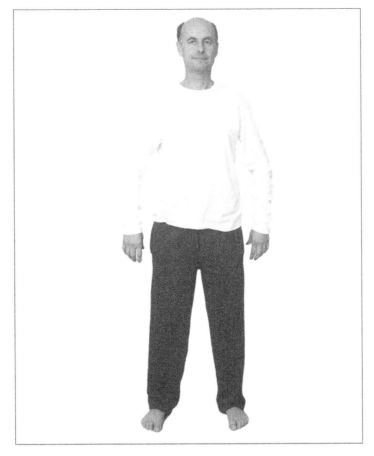

Standing posture

heels or toes of your feet. Experiment with this so that you can feel the difference between being off balance i.e. on your toes or heels, and being evenly balanced over the whole of your feet.

Sitting version

A dining room table chair or a desk chair is best. A chair that you won't sink into. Sit towards the edge of the chair so that you are supporting your own back. Now follow the instructions as for the standing version above and, even though you are sitting, develop the sensation that you are standing.

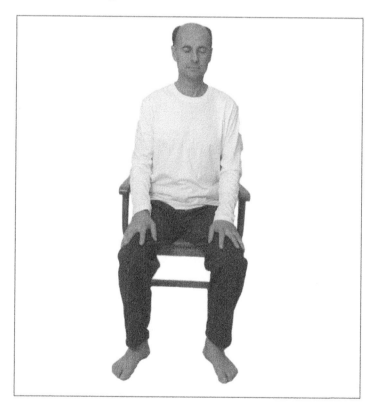

Standing posture: sitting version

Imagine that your weight is going down through your legs and through your feet, merging into the ground, just as is described in the standing instructions given above.

For both sitting and standing versions

Notice how you are breathing: are you breathing from the upper chest; from the belly; shallowly; deeply? There are no rights or wrongs at this stage, just notice.

Become aware of your perineum. This is the area of muscle between your anus and your genitals. This is not an area that we think about very much, but a very important area. Make sure your perineum is relaxed and 'open'. Have the sensation that from your perineum the rest of the torso can be lifted. Imagine a balloon being inflated which has the effect of lifting and straightening the spine. The belly however remains soft and loose and going down.

Shoulders relaxed.

Arms by your sides, palms facing backwards, or on your thighs if sitting.

Jaw loose.

Take a deep breath.

Let out some yawns or sighs. Then some sounds, 'o' (as in 'orange') is a good sound to get everything moving, try and get it to vibrate all your cells, right down to your feet.

Belly stays loose.

Flex your feet, gently bending and stretching at the toes and ankles.

Then place feet flat on the floor.

Become aware of the underside of your feet.

Feel how they contact with the floor.

Notice how you are breathing now, any difference to before?

With the next breath in, let your belly fill up, let the sides of your midriff fill up, let your back fill up.

Let the breath go right down into your hips.

From now on, whenever you have a moment to notice, allow your breath to come down into your belly. Not forcing, just allowing.

If you are sitting, develop the sensation that you are standing.

Imagine there is a little door on the underside of your right foot. When you feel ready to breathe in, let the door open and let something come in. Let the underside of your foot receive something from the earth.

What happens to your breathing?

Close the door again, any difference to your breathing?

Alternate the foot, which does the door opening, left foot, right foot, left foot, etc.

Experiment with different amounts of pressure between your foot and the floor; push down more firmly with one foot, then the other. Find the amount of pressure which feels right for you.

What happens to your breathing? It deepens?

As a last experiment, try that 'o' sound again, try it with the doors in your feet closed and then open. Any difference? With the doors open it should sound a bit more resonant, like the sound is going right through you and into the earth.

From now on, whenever you are sitting or standing, wherever you are, try and encourage that sense of connection between your feet and the earth. In qigong terms you are allowing yourself to be nourished by the energy of the earth. Just as a tree draws its strength up through its roots, so you can be strengthened, by allowing a firmer connection between your feet and the earth. Doing this exercise daily will help your legs and feet and whole body to become stronger, more vibrant, more alive.

Connecting with the energy all around you

It's not really a matter of 'doing' something, it's more an attitude of letting something happen. The flow of energy between our bodies and the surrounding environment is something, which happens naturally for children and animals. It's just that as adults we go through stresses and strains, which result in us blocking, or holding on to our natural flow.

So if you haven't noticed any relationship between the opening up of your feet, your breathing and the energy around you, don't worry, it's not that you are doing anything wrong, it's just a matter of sitting back and allowing it to happen, and then one day, it will.

Refining the posture

When you feel familiar with the guidelines above then it is time to make a couple of refinements to your posture. The aim of the refinements is to give you a well-developed awareness of what it feels like when your body is properly aligned.

When your body is out of alignment then your energy easily becomes blocked or leaks out. Good posture is therefore a fundamental first step in qigong and a fundamental first step on the path to health.

EXERCISE 9: HEAD AND NECK

Check your knees are bent, belly is soft, shoulders relaxed and spine is rising, as if lifted from the perineum.

Now turn your attention to your head. Where are you looking? Slightly down; slightly up; to one side? Most of us have a habitual gaze which is slightly off centre, as though we are trying to avoid looking at that which is right in front of us. In qigong you have to take that step, and face the world straight on.

Eyes horizontal (so if you were to draw a line out from your eyes, that line would be parallel with the floor).

Looking straight ahead, not to the right or the left. Look in a mirror to check you really are 'square on'.

Turn your attention to the place where your skull joins your neck. Is there any sense of pressure or compression there? Experiment with moving your head forwards and backwards. Find the place which feels most free of pressure. This should be when your skull is balanced evenly above your neck. Check in the mirror again or ask someone else for feedback.

Now, keeping your awareness at that point, see if you can allow your skull to lift slightly off the last vertebra of the neck. As with all qigong exercises, you are not forcing something to happen, but allowing it to happen.

Allowing your skull just to lift slightly, and allowing this lift to take place creates a space for your energy to circulate more freely. With your energy comes blood, oxygen, nutrients and healing.

As you allow your skull to rise, make sure your belly stays loose and let your hips just 'roll under', as though you are pointing your tailbone (the last few vertebrae) down to the floor.

Summary of stage 3 postures

Just check you've got everything right so far:

Feet parallel, shoulder width apart.
Knees slightly bent.
Weight going through centre of knees into centre of foot.
Perineum relaxed and open.
Spine rising, lifted from perineum.
Shoulders relaxed.
Arms by sides, palms facing backwards or on thighs if sitting.
Head straight.
Eyes horizontal.
Skull lifted off neck.
Belly soft and going down.
Hips rolled under.
Tailbone perpendicular to floor.

Relaxing into the posture

Now keep in the aligned posture, and try to relax into it. It may feel a little uncomfortable at first, but that's just because you are using your muscles in a different way. If standing, most people say that it makes them feel the muscles in the thighs to start with. That's because many people do not usually use the muscles in their thighs, instead they are used to standing with the knees 'locked' and the legs rigid, and so the thigh muscles have nothing to do but waste away.

Experiment with deliberately moving to that rigid, knees locked, way of standing and see what happens. You'll probably notice your breathing becomes 'held', i.e. shallower. Relaxed deep breathing promotes energy, blood, oxygen and nutrients. As you move back into the knees bent posture, the breath becomes deeper and more relaxed. Relaxed deep breathing brings healing.

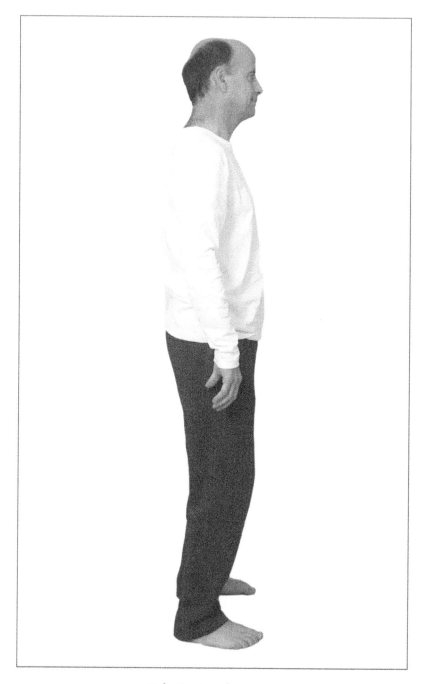

Relaxing into the posture

If you are sitting do the above exercise 'as if' you were standing, i.e. in your imagination.

Now just try and relax into your posture and let your breath deepen. Do not force your breathing to change; let it change. Let a long breath out, then do nothing, just pause, just wait, sooner or later, a breath will flow in, all by itself. Remember those doors in the bottom of your feet, let them open. It may feel as if the breath comes in through your feet as well as through your nose. If so, that's good because that's the energy of the earth merging with the energy of your body.

As the breath comes in, let it come in as much as it's needed. Let the muscles in your belly and chest fully relax, so that they can expand as much as they need. Then, let go of the breath completely. Let out as much breath as possible, then just wait, do not pull or suck in the breath, relax and wait till the breath comes flowing in, all by itself.

The out-breath should not cause your body to sag at all. The out-breath can be invigorating, leaving each cell freshly washed, freshly energized. You will find it helpful, when breathing out, to raise the soft palate of the mouth. The soft palate is on the roof of the mouth, just to the rear of the hard section. The soft palate is raised when you make the 'o' sound as in orange. You can do this silently, just imaging you are about to say 'orange'. Raising the soft palate on the out-breath helps to make the exhalation an invigorating process rather than a sagging process.

Whilst focusing on your breathing, you may find it helpful to bring the memory of the sea to mind. Remember how the sea flows in and flows out again, very relaxed yet unstoppable. So it is with the energy of the breath, and behind that, the energy of the universe. Relaxed yet unstoppable. Yet, we do try to stop it, by bracing ourselves, by tightening our muscles, by holding on. Qigong is about letting go, and through letting go, finding enormous strength.

A final reminder concerning this exercise and tai chi/qigong in general: **letting go does not mean collapsing.**

The posture you are learning establishes a vital framework through which energy can flow. You are not a sandbag on the beach, which the sea passes over. You are more like the dolphin whose supple frame is invigorated with each current.

Stage 4: Self-healing – creating inner space

When you feel comfortable with the aligned posture of stage 3 and comfortable with your breathing, it is time to start dissolving inner tension or 'blocks' and creating some inner space so that healing can take place.

EXERCISE 10: CREATING INNER SPACE

Have another stretch and shake, try allowing your whole body to shake a bit, like a dog shaking itself after it's got wet.

Now, whether sitting or standing, come back to the initial posture you cultivated previously.

Tune in to your body. Which part of your body feels uncomfortable? It may be a feeling of tightness or a feeling of weakness or numbness. If it is easily contactable, you may find it helpful to place your hand on that area. What does it feel like under your hand? As you tune in to the area, which feels uncomfortable, does a colour come to you? Or a sensation? Does the discomfort have a shape to it?

Allow those sensations or colours or shapes to be there. As you breathe in, imagine you are breathing in to that area. As you breathe out, imagine you are allowing more space to be created there.

Allow all the muscle fibres around that area to become longer and broader, and in so doing allowing any bones near that area (including vertebrae), to space apart.

As you allow an inner letting go then 'something' is released. That something may be something physical like muscle tension, or it may be some form of held emotion. You may feel a wave of sadness or anger, you may even feel a wave of laughter. Whatever was not allowed in the past became held in the body, and you are now giving it space to be released.

Have a general attitude of letting go down towards the floor. Just notice the emotions come and go, notice the muscle tension change as sensations come and go and move towards the floor.

Helping everything move down

EXERCISE 11: THE TAI CHI STARTING PATTERN

Once you have created some inner space it is useful to bring in a movement. This is a movement which helps to move the released tension down towards the floor and also which encourages a sense of being re-charged with fresh 'chi'. The movement is often called the 'tai chi starting pattern'. This is because it is often used at the start of many tai chi forms and also because it encompasses many of the initial skills that one is trying to develop in tai chi. The movement is, at first sight, quite simple. However, as with many tai chi/qigong movements, it can be entered into with many different levels of awareness. The movement is conventionally performed standing; however if you cannot stand for very long, or if standing is too un-comfortable, it can also be carried out sitting. The sitting version will be described first.

Sitting version

A kitchen or dining chair is best. Try and sit on the edge of the chair so that your spine can lengthen and you are not slumping into the back of the chair. Make sure your feet are planted firmly on the ground. Try and feel how the up and down movement of your arms symbolizes a movement of energy right through your legs too. In this way your legs can also become suffused with the fresh chi.

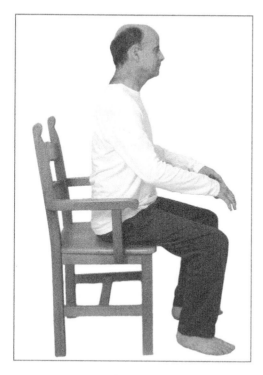

The tai chi starting pattern: sitting version

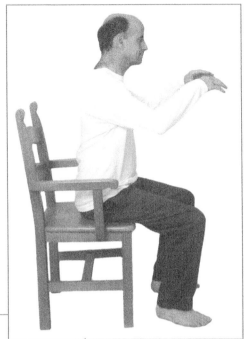

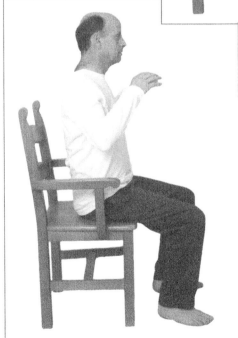

The tai chi starting pattern: sitting version

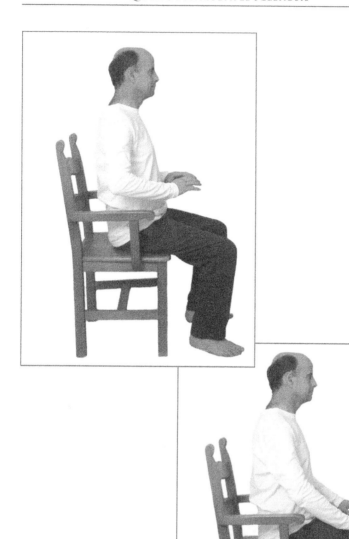

The tai chi starting pattern: sitting version (continued)

Allow both arms to rise. The word 'allow' is very important here. It is not as if you are yanking your arms up. It is more as if your arms are being lifted, by some unseen force. The elbows are soft and slightly bent. The hands and wrists are soft, and so follow along, slightly behind the movement of the arms. Breathe in as the arms are ascending. Have a sense that your body is being nourished by energy rising up from the ground beneath your feet.

Allow the arms to come up to just below shoulder height. The wrists then come in towards the body, and the arms begin their downward journey. As the arms go down, allow any tension from your body to flow down towards your feet and out into the earth. Let everything go to a place deep in the earth. See Appendix for a reminder of the process of grounding and contacting the nurturing energy of the earth.

Standing version

Firstly broaden your stance. This should be accomplished by shifting your weight to one leg, and stepping out to one side with the other leg.

Allow both arms to rise. The word 'allow' is very important here. It is not as if you are yanking your arms up. It is more as if your arms are being lifted, by some unseen force. The elbows are soft and slightly bent. The hands and wrists are soft, and so follow along, slightly behind the movement of the arms. Breathe in as the arms are ascending.

Allow the arms to come up to just below shoulder height. The wrists then come in towards the body, and the arms begin their downward journey. At the same time the knees slightly bend, and you start to breathe out.

On the downward movement your weight shifts slightly back on to the heels and you allow a sense of letting your inner tension release towards the floor. Sense how you can let go to a place beneath your feet, deep into the earth.

At the lowest point of the downward movement, shift your weight slightly forward on to the ball of the foot. This activates an acupressure point called 'the bubbling spring', which, as the name suggests, allows for fresh energy to be taken up from the ground into the body.

As you breathe in, sense how that fresh energy can be absorbed by all your tissues, nerves and blood.

For both sitting and standing versions

Repeat the cycle of up and down numerous times, releasing old 'negative chi' and re-charging with fresh 'positive chi'. I won't say how many times because that depends on your individual ability to sit or stand and to focus in this way. Be guided by your own body and your own feelings. Let your body tell you when the process is complete.

At the end of the exercise, pause. Let your hands rest over the lower dantien. Breathe down into the dantien. Breathe out from the dantien. Let your breathing be relaxed. You may find yourself moving or juddering or shaking, that's fine and is just a sign that you are still releasing tension. As you release the tension from an area of your body so you allow that part of yourself to become more fully alive. Enjoy that feeling of becoming more fully alive. Allow any sensations to come and go like waves. Continue sitting or standing until you feel ready to move into the next set of exercises, involving balance and walking.

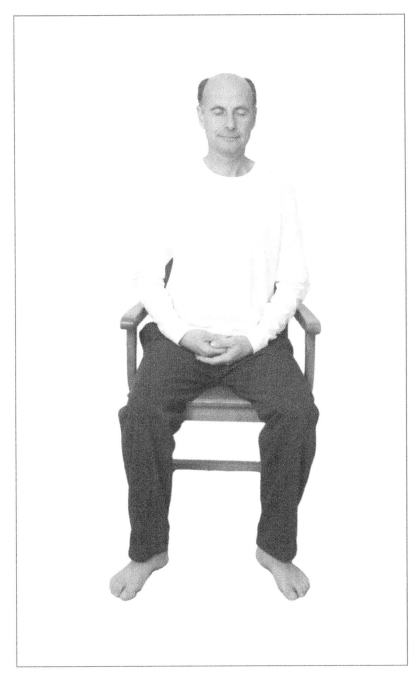

The tai chi starting pattern: end of the exercise

Chapter 6

Qigong Exercises: Developing Balance and Finding your Feet Again

My level of fatigue has reduced and I do not feel as unsteady.
(Comment from participant in the research study)

This chapter will initially take you through two ways of improving your balance. Once your balance has improved, then it will be time to put your new found balance into practice with a special exercise to help you walk more stably and fluidly.

Stage 5: Developing a sense of balance

If you have been sitting up till now, now is the time to stand. This exercise strengthens the legs and energizes the entire body but the benefits of this exercise can only really be gained from a standing position. If you have difficulty in standing, you may like to stand in front of a desk or table. You can then lightly rest your fingers on the table if you feel you are losing balance.

EXERCISE 12: PREPARATION FOR MOVEMENT

Adopt the same standing posture as described in Chapter 5, stage 3.

Shift your weight over to the right leg so that you can then raise the left foot, so that only the ball of the foot is in contact with the floor.

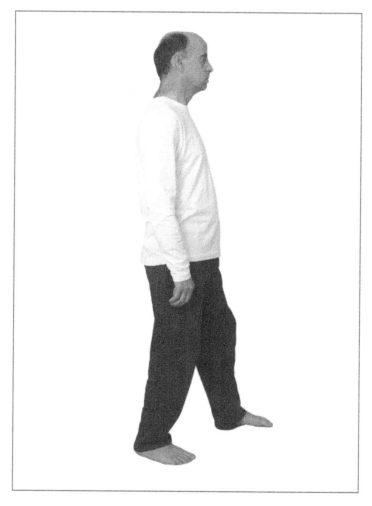

Preparation for movement

Bring your left foot forward with the heel striking the floor first and then roll the weight forward on to the left foot. Both feet should now be facing forwards in a parallel position. The feet should be approximately shoulder width apart.

Imagine a vertical line that goes through your nose, sternum, navel and perineum (area between your anus and genitals) and goes down to the floor. This vertical line should be kept straight and perpendicular to the floor. Don't go wonky!

Check that your knees are slightly bent, that your hips are rolled under, your belly is soft and that your head is held lightly on your neck.

Take your time; the next exercise should be done quite slowly to start with. In Exercise 13 below, when your weight comes over one leg, pause, then take a moment to feel how your weight goes through that leg, into your foot and into the floor. Try to sense what it would be like if you had roots coming out of that foot, and going into the floor. This isn't an exercise of imagination, it is rather an exercise in extending sensation and sensory awareness, below your foot into the floor.

In Exercise 13, you will be shifting your weight and thereby encouraging the flow of energy up and down each side of your body. As you shift your weight over one leg, energy goes down that leg and into the earth. As you move your weight onto the other leg, energy is drawn up your first leg to circulate round the body and then down into the new weighted leg.

When you do Exercise 13, move very slowly, let your breathing be very relaxed and just be aware of your own experience of energy and breath.

EXERCISE 13: LEARNING TO SHIFT
BALANCE BACKWARDS AND FORWARDS

You are now going to get used to the idea of shifting your weight from the back leg to the front leg several times. When shifting the weight forwards your knee should never go over your toes. Thus you should always be able to see your toes. If your knee covers your toes then you are more likely to lose balance and topple forwards. The knees of both legs should be slightly bent at all times. At no point should either leg become locked or rigid.

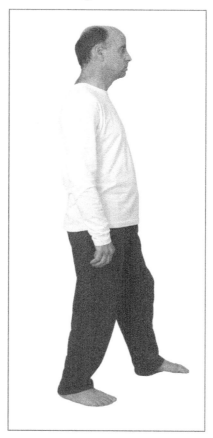

Shifting balance backwards and forwards

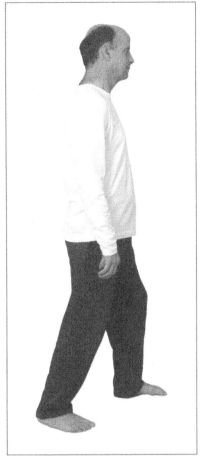

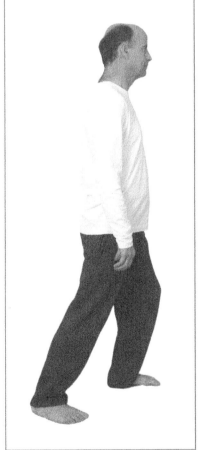

Shifting balance backwards and forwards

Very slowly, and in your own time, get used to the idea of gently shifting weight forwards on to the front foot and then shifting the weight back on to the back foot. Bring your awareness down to your feet. As you breathe in be aware of the contact of each foot with the floor. As you breathe out, imagine you are extending that contact deeper down towards the centre of the earth. As you breathe in you are breathing in from the centre of the earth and as you breathe out, you are breathing down to the centre of the earth.

Imagine a line coming out of your perineum extending down to the floor and below the floor into the earth. Feel how, as you move backwards and forwards, you are also moving this line through the earth beneath your feet, backwards and forwards. By carrying out this aspect of the exercise in your imagination you will be encouraging your sense of connection with the ground, deepening your stability and improving your balance and making you less vulnerable to falling.

EXERCISE 14: BRINGING THE ARMS INTO THE MOVEMENT

When you feel you have mastered the first stage of this exercise, that of shifting weight backwards and forwards, you may then like to progress to the second stage which is to bring the arms into the movement.

As you shift your weight forward on to the left leg, bring your right elbow up so it is level with the bottom of your ribcage.

The forearm should then become parallel with the floor.

As you move forward on to the left leg, the right hand extends as if pushing open a door.

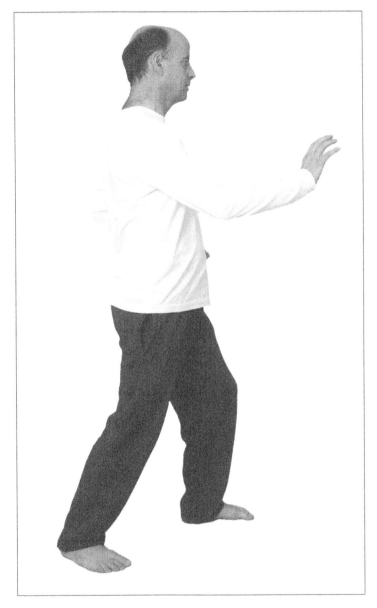

Involving the right arm

As you shift your weight back on to the right leg, the right hand comes back with the movement of the body as though pulling on a rope.

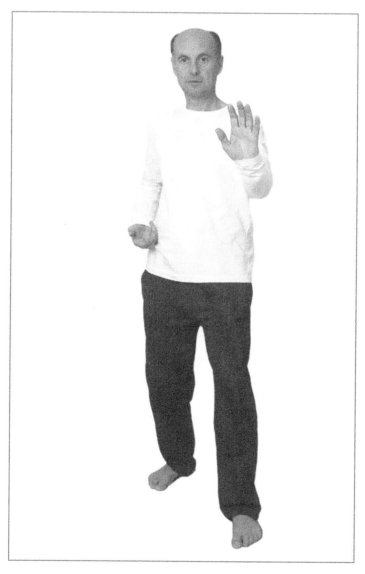

Involving the left arm

When you feel you have fluidly incorporated the right arm into the movement, you may then like to bring the left arm into the movement. The left arm does the opposite of whatever the right arm is doing.

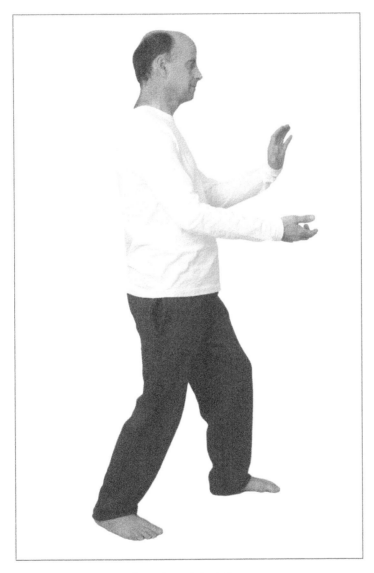

The right and the left arms

Thus when the right arm is going forward, the left arm is pulling back on the imaginary rope. When the right arm is pulling back on the imaginary rope, the left arm is pushing forward on the imaginary door.

This exercise is excellent as a foundation for improving confidence in shifting your balance forwards and backwards. It is therefore an excellent preparation for the next set of exercises in this chapter concerned with the movements of walking.

Stage 6: Finding your feet again

Visualize a tiger walking slowly and you will find that your steps become as majestic as his. (Thich Nhat Hanh 1996)

When working with people with multiple sclerosis (MS), I usually ask them to take a few steps so that I can see how they are walking. Many people with MS suffer from the phenomenon of 'dropped foot'. This means that the first connection with the ground is made by the toes instead of the heel. This method of walking does not provide sufficient stability and falls or loss of balance often results. Some people with MS also have the tendency to throw themselves forward with the upper body and the legs get pulled along behind. This also has the problem of making falls and loss of balance more likely. When learning to walk in this balanced way, it is vital that the heel is the first part of the foot to make contact with the floor. Second, there should be a rolling through the foot onto the ball of the foot and lastly, onto the toes. The toes are often forgotten about, but are very important in giving a sense of propulsion as the foot leaves the floor. Learning to walk in qigong fashion is best attempted without shoes. When walking barefoot, one can really feel how the foot makes contact with the floor.

One of the most important things is to slow down. You're not in a rush to get anywhere, your only aim is to bring your awareness into your body, so that your awareness can inhabit your body in a clear, focused way.

Roger Jahnke (2002) describes this as follows: 'You're walking but the destination is not a place, it is a state – the qigong state' (p.46).

The Buddhist monk, Thich Nhat Hanh has written a wonderful guide to walking meditation called 'The Long Road Turns to Joy' (1996). His book includes the following recommendations:

> When you begin to practise walking meditation, you might feel unbalanced, like a baby learning to walk… Visualize a tiger walking slowly and you will find that your steps become as majestic as his.

We're not used to thinking about walking as being a path to spiritual enlightenment; however, Thich Nhat Hanh relates a story when the Buddha was asked:

> 'What do you and your disciples practise?' and he replied, 'We sit, we walk and we eat.' The questioner continued, 'But sir, everyone sits, walks and eats.' The Buddha told him, 'When we sit, we know we are sitting. When we walk, we know we are walking. When we eat, we know we are eating.'

Thich Nhat Hanh goes on to say: 'To have peace you can begin by walking peacefully. Everything depends on your steps' (pp.4–5).

So how can we translate these fine words into action?

Qigong walking

Qigong walking encourages a lower centre of gravity than we would experience in normal walking. This adds to stability and improves balance. One way to encourage a lower centre of gravity is to avoid the inclination to lift your body as you step. You will then become aware that you have to use the muscles of your thighs to propel yourself forward. You are thus minimizing the 'bobbing' up and down of normal walking.

Finding your feet again also requires slowing the whole process down. In the section below are some useful moment-by-moment instructions to help you regain control over your walking, improve your balance and move towards a sense of peace.

EXERCISE 15: FINDING YOUR FEET AGAIN: MOMENT-BY-MOMENT

Take on the aligned posture that we developed in Chapter 5. Remember to cultivate the feeling of the spine being lengthened as if extended from above by a piece of thread attached to the top of the head.

Remember also that the belly should stay soft so the feeling of lengthening is up the back of the body and the feeling of softening goes down the front of the body.

Shift your weight onto your right leg. This frees up the left leg, so it is ready to step forward.

Have the sense that you're dropping your tailbone towards the floor and step forward on your left foot, but keep your weight on the back leg. Make sure that the heel of the foot connects with the ground first of all.

Keep both legs still but transfer your weight to the left leg so that your weight rolls forward towards the centre of the foot. As you move your weight forward imagine that the movement takes place underground as well as above ground.

Keep your body in the same low position and when the right leg feels released step forward, again ensuring the heel of the foot makes contact with the floor first. Do not transfer your weight to the leading foot until your body weight is over the centre of the foot.

As you move forward with each step keep your body weight, and thus your centre of gravity, low. Imagine the tailbone connecting to the floor, feeling how the foot rolls with each step, noticing how the movement of each step goes right through to the toes and the toes aid in the propulsion forward.

You need to practise the above movements for a considerable time before they become second nature, as Thich Nhat Hanh stated in the quote above. You may initially 'feel unbalanced, like a baby learning to walk'.

However, after some time you will find that the movements become natural and you will wonder why you ever walked in your old unbalanced fashion.

Benefits

The above exercise, although in some ways quite simple, can have remarkable benefits. The improved confidence that comes with knowing you're not likely to fall over leads to further confidence in carrying out a range of activities. Also slowing down your mind and your attention so that you really bring your attention into the process of walking can be an important first step towards being fully present in the here and now.

Stage 7: Meditation – gathering and centring

At the end of your daily qigong exercise programme it is very useful to have a closing exercise. The closing exercise simply encourages you to gather your energy together and come to a feeling of being 'centred'. As I have described previously, in qigong (as in tai chi and yoga and the martial arts) the main energy centre of the body, the lower dantien, is just below the navel.

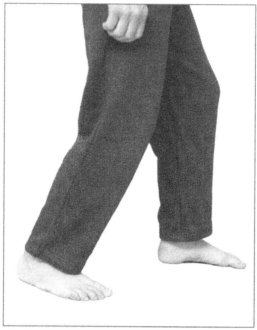

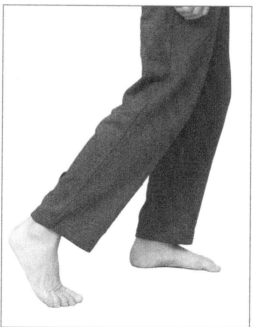

Finding your feet again

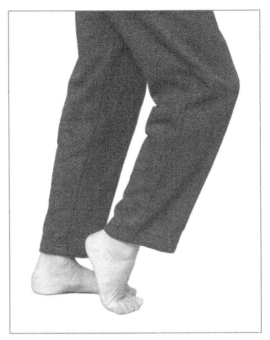

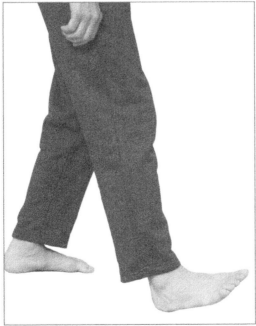

Finding your feet again

EXERCISE 16: GATHERING AND CENTRING YOUR ENERGY

Sit down on the edge of a chair so that you are supporting your own back, as described in Exercise 1. Place your hands in your lap as though you were 'cupping' the area below your navel.

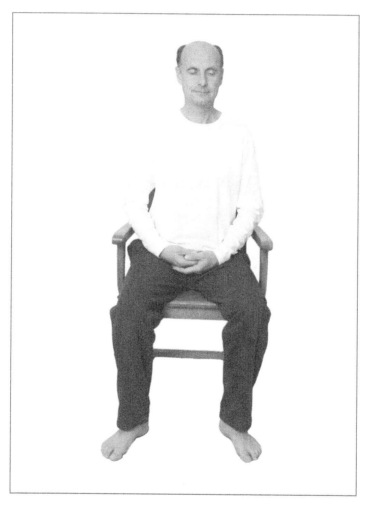

Gathering and centring

Imagine that your energy can come to rest at this place. This is the spring from which your energy flows and it is also the reservoir where your energy is stored.

Close your eyes; let your breath go down to the lower dantien. Feel as though this is the place where you breathe from and breathe to. Initially you may find it useful to count each breath. When you first commence your training programme you may find that ten breaths down to the lower dantien is enough, before your mind starts to wander. As you progress you will find that your ability to stay in the moment and your ability to accompany your breath increases.

When your body and mind tell you that you have done enough for today, congratulate yourself on having completed your qigong sequence, congratulate yourself on taking another step towards ownership of your body and congratulate yourself on having taken another step towards health.

Chapter 7

How to Cope
with Stress

As mentioned in Chapter 4, there is some well-validated research, which shows that people with MS are more likely to suffer a relapse after the experience of a trauma or stressful event (Buljevac *et al.* 2003; Golan *et al.* 2008).

Furthermore, some people with MS describe how when they bring to mind a previous trauma they notice a tendency for their symptoms to momentarily worsen.

You will remember how I explained previously that bringing to mind the memory of a trauma activates your sympathetic nervous system. It is as though your nervous system thinks that the threat of the trauma is still present. Your nervous system is, in effect, preparing you for action against a threat, which is no longer there. Sympathetic arousal is not good for an already overactive immune system. If you can learn to reduce your nervous tension, then your immune system is more likely to come into balance and your body is less likely to tip into another relapse.

Creating a safe place in your mind

This approach involves reminding your nervous system, and your body in general, of a state of safety that you have previously experienced. This 'reminding' needs to take place not just as a mental exercise, but as a whole body and mind process.

Just as the fear of your MS has activated a state of 'danger', which has got stuck, so it is also possible to activate a state of 'safety' and to continually dip into that safety so that the state of danger becomes more manageable, more survivable.

It is not that you can simply swap danger for safety. Unfortunately it is not that simple. It is more a process of developing a sense that you can allow yourself to experience the danger whilst still feeling supported by your sense of inner safety.

Different people have different ways into safety. I have already described some physical ways of helping your body to feel safe in Chapters 5 and 6. In addition to these physical methods, some people also find it useful to cultivate images that access a feeling of safety.

Images

An image of safety needs to bring with it a whole lot of sensations and body memories of being safe. In effect the image triggers the whole nervous system, including the limbic system, to shift out of hyper- or hypoarousal and into a different mode.

The image may be an actual memory. For example one lady I worked with was a church organist, and, for her, the memory of sitting in the church and playing the organ brought with it a total body feeling of 'being in the middle of a ball of light that protected [her] from everything'.

Some people find it difficult to come up with an actual memory that makes them feel safe or protected. However they may find that they can create an image which does the same job.

For example one gentleman I worked with came up with the image of being in a lighthouse, with very thick walls and his attention was focused on keeping the light glowing (in this case it was an old-fashioned oil lamp which needed tending), whilst the storm (i.e. his trauma) raged outside the lighthouse. There are two useful things about this image. First, he feels safe inside, and comfortable in the knowledge that the storm must eventually pass, as all storms do. Second, the direction of his attention is towards keeping the light glowing.

When he initially worked with this image he put himself on the balcony of the lighthouse, shouting at the darkening clouds and trying to fight the storm, which was exhausting and put him still very much in 'hyperarousal mode'. It was only when he shifted his attention to cultivating the inner light that the beneficial effects of his image began to work. He noticed that the light became brighter and brighter until it filled his attention and the storm became just a faint tapping on the window, which he was quite content to let tap away.

Whatever image you use, it is hoped that you will find a sense of increased spaciousness. Spaciousness is one of the most important qualities that is required for energy to flow and for healing to take place.

Flashbacks

'Flashbacks' are when you see a traumatic event that you went through, happening again. For some people the flashback is not so much a picture, as a replay of the sounds or even smells that were around at the time of the incident.

Flashbacks often take you back to the worst moment of the incident, maybe the moment when you thought you were going to die or something bad was about to happen. It is as though your mind hasn't quite come to terms with what happened and needs to go back there and understand it again.

Flashbacks often bring up the same thoughts or feelings that were around at that worst moment. So you may again have the thought, 'I am going to die' and you may again experience a wave of panic or terror.

It is as though part of your mind is still frozen at that moment in time and somehow has not been updated to the fact that you came through this experience and you survived.

COPING WITH FLASHBACKS

One of the best ways of coping with flashbacks is to do a sort of 'updating' procedure. A computer analogy would be that the software is out of date and somehow you need to update it. This process is described below:

1. As way of preparation think about a time towards the end of your traumatic incident, when you knew that the worst was over and that you had come through it. This may be a time when you literally let out a breath and said something to yourself like, 'well that was really bad, but I came through it'.

    It may be that your trauma left you in a lot of pain, or you were traumatized by what happened to someone else, and it may be that you are still living with that physical or emotional pain now. In that case you need to find a time when something of that physical or emotional pain subsided.

    For some people this is when they arrived at hospital and felt they could relax a little, when they knew they were getting medical attention. For other people it may not have been till they were discharged from hospital and arrived back at their own house or some 'place of safety'. For some people this point may have been minutes after the 'worst moment', for others it may be hours, days or even weeks.

2. Now you are going to imagine that the experience of your trauma is like a video or a short film. The point you have established in point 1 above, is the end of the video. It is very important to have this end point firmly

established. Your mind needs to know that the worst moment of the trauma had some sort of end.

3.   Now, when a flashback occurs what do you normally do? Most people try and distract themselves, turn the TV on, make a cup of tea. This is OK, except that it leaves your nervous system activated and in the middle of the worst bit, that is, re-traumatized. You need to remind both your body and your mind that there was an ending to this 'worst bit'. You need to remind your body and mind of the end point which you have established.

4.   So, after the flashback of the worst moment has occurred, keep the video going. Keep it going right through till the end point you have established.

5.   It may be that the flashback has left you feeling so overwhelmed that you do not feel able to do this straight away. In that case give yourself a few minutes, carry out the qigong grounding exercises and enter the safe place we established earlier. Then, when you feel sufficiently resourced, start from where the flashback finished and then take the video through to the end point.

6.   When you get to the end point, allow yourself to breathe out and then choose one of the 'creating safety' exercises described earlier. You will remember these include: the 'grounding' exercise on p.54; the safe place 'images' exercise on p.106 and the 'light stream' exercise on p.57.

7.   Well done, you have taken a very important step in overcoming trauma. This process may have to be repeated again and again, and each time you do it your body and mind is being reassured that that moment has passed now. You are here now.

8. So take a look around, remind yourself of the date and the time that it is NOW; remind yourself where you are. Notice the colours of your surroundings, notice what sounds you can hear. Bring yourself back to the sensation of the ground under your feet.

9. OK, what do you need to do right now? If you are still feeling agitated, the negative chi which has been released needs to move more thoroughly through your body.

Moving the trauma through your body

It may feel like your body is still somehow 'holding' the trauma. You may notice your heart rate is still higher than usual, you may feel more sweaty than usual. You may feel that your stomach is churning with the anxiety. If so, it can be useful to go through the stretching and shaking exercises described in Chapter 5. Imagine how the nervous tension is leaving your body. Feel how the tension can be shaken out of your fingertips and how it can also leave your body through the soles of your feet and soak away into the earth. When you feel the inner tension has been released somewhat, then repeat the safe place exercises described above.

Chapter 8

Putting it Into Practice and Taking it Further

On waking

Put on the kettle!

Prepare a mug of herbal tea or warm water with lemon. Sip at intervals throughout the morning qigong session. Top up as needed.

Carry out:

Creating safety exercise.

Stretching and bouncing exercises.

Alignment exercises.

Self-healing.

Shifting balance exercises.

Walking exercise.

Closing meditation.

In between the morning and evening formal practice sessions, there is a large chunk of time! This time should not be spent ignoring all the principles you have been trying to cultivate in the formal sessions. Throughout the day there are many, many opportunities to put the qigong principles into practice. Try and generally make your movements softer and more full of a gentle awareness. Be aware of your posture and breathing. Allow yourself to feel supported by the 'chi' around you.

Just before going to bed

Carry out:

> Creating safety exercise.
>
> Alignment exercise.
>
> Self-healing exercise.
>
> Shifting balance exercise.
>
> Walking exercise.
>
> Closing meditation.

Sleep well, breathe well, heal well.

Taking it further

You can deepen your practice of qigong and thus increase its effectiveness in several ways:

- Read some books about qigong. I would particularly recommend the texts by Jahnke (2002) and Frantzis (2007). Both of these authors also have instructional DVDs which can be purchased from their websites (see details in Useful Websites).

- Obtain some instructional DVDs or CDs. I would again particularly recommend the above authors. Their websites are provided at the end of this book.

- If you are following instructional material from a book, CD, or DVD you need to make sure you keep within the limits of what feels safe for you. Do not attempt or persist with any exercise that feels it is putting you at risk of falling, or otherwise hurting yourself. Respect your instinct.

- Find an instructor. Qigong is most effectively learnt through 'live' instruction. This book is intended as a complement to such live instruction. An instructor can see if you are encountering any problems or implementing incorrect practice. The websites at the end of this book give details of instructors in many countries throughout the world.

- It is important to note that there are many different types of qigong. For people with multiple sclerosis (MS) I would recommend what is often referred to as the 'water approach'. This refers to a type of instruction, which advocates softening and flowing. The opposite approach is often called the fire approach. This uses more forceful breathing and vigorous techniques, which would not be so appropriate for people with MS. You need to find an instructor who is used to adapting his or her traditional teaching so that it can be carried out by someone with a disability. I would suggest you ask to observe a class first and see if you feel you could manage the exercises being given. Many qigong instructors are happy to give individualized one-to-one instruction, which could then be adapted to your individual needs.

GROUNDING AND BREATHING

This exercise is to help you feel more secure in your body so you can cope with difficult feelings or the sense of stress as it comes upon you. Most of the time when we feel stressed, it is a sense as though our energy is coming up to the head and everything is buzzing and feeling out of control. So in grounding we try and encourage the opposite, which is a sense that our energy can go down towards the ground, literally down to the earth beneath our feet. The first step is to develop a posture which is going to encourage this sense of grounding and encourage a sense of safety in your body. It is good to use a hard-backed chair and to sit slightly forward in the chair and then to have a sense that there is a piece of string attached to the top of your head, which is just going to lift your spine slightly. Keep the belly soft so that you can breathe easily. This gives a sense that the back of the body is being lengthened, going up towards the sky. The front of your body is softening and going down. Make sure your shoulders are relaxed and make sure your head feels loose and just suspended on top of your spine. Allow yourself to breathe freely. As you breathe in, just be aware of any tension across the chest and as you breathe out, just let it go. Let a longer breath out than usual and as you breathe out, imagine something like a wave coming down your arms and out through your fingertips.

If you feel any sense of distress, it's good to have the idea that this distress can leave your body first, down the arms and out through the fingers and second, down the legs and out through the feet. Practise this now, so as you breathe in, just be aware of any uncomfortable feelings in your body. Breathe in and let go, and as you breathe out, just let those unwanted feelings pass down the arms and out through the fingertips. Let's bring your attention to a lower part of the body. If you have uncomfortable feelings in your belly area and stomach, then it's generally easier to let go of these down through the legs. So as you breathe in, just be aware of how it feels in your belly. As you breathe out, just let go of any unwanted feelings down the legs and out through the feet into the floor.

It is important that your feet are flat on the floor, and that the soles of your feet have a sense of melting and merging into the ground beneath the building you are in. You may even find it useful to imagine roots going deep down from your feet, deep into the earth. Just as a tree has roots, which extend down into the earth as much as a tree extends above the earth, so imagine that you too can have roots of awareness which are almost doing the same thing as roots from a tree. The roots are trying to dig down in between stones, seeking out moisture, seeking out nutrients from deep in the soil. So as you breathe in, notice how it feels in your body. As you breathe out, let any unwanted feelings pass down your legs and down through those roots deep into the earth beneath your feet, letting the earth soak up the unwanted distress.

REFERENCES

Beinfield, H. and Korngold, E. (1991) *Between Heaven and Earth. A Guide to Chinese Medicine.* New York: Ballantine.

Buckley, T. (2007) *The Multiple Sclerosis Diet Book.* London: Sheldon Press.

Buljevac, D., Hop, W.C., Reedeker, W., Janssens, A.C., Van der Meche, F.G., Van Doorn, P.A. and Hintzen, R.Q. (2003) 'Self reported stressful life events and exacerbation in multiple sclerosis.' *British Medical Journal 327*, 646.

Capra, F. (1991) *The Tao of Physics: An Exploration of the Parallels between Modern Physics and Eastern Mysticism.* Boston, MA: Shambhala.

Clark, A. (2000) *The Complete Illustrated Guide to Tai Chi.* London: Element.

Fleming, N. (2007) 'Warning on wi-fi health risk to children.' *Daily Telegraph,* 28 April 2007.

Frantzis, B.K. (1993, 2007) *Opening the Energy Gates of Your Body. Gain Life-long Vitality.* Berkeley, CA: North Atlantic Books.

Golan, D., Somer, E. and Dishon, S. (2008) 'Impact of exposure to war stress on exacerbation in multiple sclerosis.' *Annals of Neurology 64*, 2, 143–148.

Hua-Ching, N. (1993) *Life and Teachings of Two Immortals (Vol. 1).* Santa Monica, CA: Seven Star Communications.

Jacobson, B., Ho-Cheng, C., Cashel, C. and Guerro, L. (1997) 'The effect of tai chi on balance, kinaesthetic sense and strength.' *Perceptual Motor Skills 84*, 27–33.

Jahnke, J. (2002) *The Healing Promise of Qi.* San Francisco, CA: Contemporary Books.

Jelinek, G. (2005) *Taking Control of Multiple Sclerosis. Natural and Medical Therapies to Prevent its Progression.* London: Impala Books.

Joyce, N. and Richardson, R. (1997) 'Reflexology can help multiple sclerosis.' *International Journal of Alternative and Complementary Medicine*, July, 10–12.

Kabat-Zin, J. (1990) *Full Catastrophe Living; Using the Wisdom of your Body and Mind to Face Stress, Pain and Illness.* New York, NY: Delacorte.

Kabat-Zin, J., Lipworth, L., Burney, R. and Sellers, W. (1987) 'Four-year follow-up of a meditation based programme for chronic pain.' *Clinical Journal of Pain 2*, 159–173.

Kaplin, K., Goldenberg, D. and Galvin-Nadeau M. (1993) 'The impact of a meditation based programme on fibromyalgia.' *General Hospital Psychiatry 15*, 284–289.

Kaptchuk, T. (2000) *Chinese Medicine. The Web That Has No Weaver.* London: Rider.

Leggett, D. (1999) *Recipes for Self-Healing.* Totnes, UK: Meridian Press.

Levine, P. (1997) *Waking the Tiger, Healing Trauma.* Berkeley, CA: North Atlantic Books.

Mills, N. and Allen, J. (2000) 'Mindfulness of movement as a coping strategy in multiple sclerosis. A pilot study.' *General Hospital Psychiatry 22*, 425–431.

Mills, N., Allen, J. and Carey-Morgan, S. (2000) 'Does tai chi/qigong help patients with multiple sclerosis?' *Journal of Body Work and Movement Therapies 4*, 39–48.

Ni, Maoshing (1995) *The Yellow Emperor's Classic Book of Medicine.* Boston and London: Shambhala.

Nittby, H. (2008) *Effect of mobile phone radiation on the mammalian brain.* Dissertation, Department of Clinical Science, University of Lund (abstract available at www.lu.se).

Oschman, J.L. (2000) *The Scientific Basis for Energy Medicine.* London: Churchill Livingstone.

Petajan, J.H. and White, A.T. (1999) 'Recommendations for physical activity in patients with multiple sclerosis.' *Sports Medicine 27,* 179–191.

Peterson, E., Cho, C. and von Kock, L. (2008) 'Injurious falls among middle aged and older adults with multiple sclerosis.' *Physical Medicine 89,* 6, 1031–1107.

Salford, L.G., Brun, A.E., Eberhardt, J.L., Malmgren, L. and Persson, B.R.R. (2003) 'Nerve cell damage in mammalian brain after exposure to microwaves from GSM mobile phones.' *Environmental Health Perspectives,* January.

Thich Nhat Hanh (1996) *The Long Road Turns to Joy.* Berkerley, CA: Parallax Press.

Tse, S.K. and Bailey, D.M. (1992) 'Tai chi and postural control in the well elderly.' *American Journal of Occupational Therapy 46,* 295–300.

Waksman, B.K. (1994) 'Can psychoneuro-immunology help explain disease? The example of multiple sclerosis.' *Advances: The Journal of Mind-Body Health 10,* 4, 16–22.

Wolf, S., Barnhart, H., Ellision, G. and Coogler, C. (1997) 'The effect of tai chi on postural stability on older subjects.' *Physical Therapy 77,* 371–386.

Useful websites

www.nigelmillstherapies.co.uk

This is the website of the author and provides information on his therapy and classes in the South Wales area (UK).

www.takingcontrolofmultiplesclerosis.org

Provides practical information about a range of self-help strategies for people with MS.

www.mstrust.org.uk

The website of the Multiple Sclerosis Trust, which promotes research and education into MS.

www.mssociety.org.uk

The MS society is a charitable body that supports research and education for people with MS.

www.energyarts.com

Website of Bruce Frantzis; gives details of training events and instructors, mostly in the USA, although also includes details of some European training events and instructors.

www.healerwithin.com

Website of Roger Jahnke, American author of *The Healing Promise of Qi,* which gives practical guidance on some aspects of qigong as well as training events in the USA.

www.Qigong-southwest.co.uk

The website of two excellent teachers of qigong, both students of Zhixing Wang (see below), who provide training at a variety of locations throughout the south west of the UK.

www.dao-hua-Qigong.com

The website of Zhixing Wang, a very accomplished Chinese teacher of qigong, who provides regular weekend courses in London and longer retreats, mainly in the south east of the UK.

www.Qigonginstitute.org

A website that promotes research and education into qigong.

www.tcckf.org.uk

A UK website that promotes the use of tai chi and qigong for people with disabilities or special needs.

www.taichifinder.co.uk

A UK website that provides listings of tai chi and qigong classes throughout the UK. Just enter your postcode and it tells you the class nearest to you.

INDEX

CPI Antony Rowe
Eastbourne, UK
November 11, 2022